THE ULTIMATE BACKBRIDGE STRETCH BOOK

PERMISSIONS

Teachers who purchase or for whom schools purchase the complete *The Lost Tools of Writing* package are granted permission to duplicate pages from the Teacher's Guide for their personal use. They are also granted permission to copy pages from the Teacher's Guide as reference pages for their students, including, but not limited to, the assessment guides provided in this Teacher's Guide.

One Student Workbook should be purchased for each student who is taught *The Lost Tools of Writing*. Some Invention worksheets will be imitated more than once. If the teacher or student wishes to copy these pages, they may do so, but only for the individual student who possesses the Student Workbook. Students are also encouraged to imitate the pattern of the worksheet on their own paper.

Permission is not granted to copy worksheets or exercise forms or any other material from one student's workbook for other students.

Permission is granted for quotations and short excerpts to be used in published materials with the condition that the source of those quotations and excerpts is included in the published materials.

For longer excerpts, please contact us via info@circeinstitute.org.

To the many teachers and students who have provided feedback, asked questions, and studied diligently.

This program is for you and because of you.

TABLE *of* CONTENTS

REVIEW LESSON
Invention Review - 11
Arrangement Review - 13
Elocution Review - 15

JUDICIAL ADDRESS ONE
Invention: Character Bias - 19
Arrangement: Refining the Narratio - 21
Elocution A: Personification - 24
Elocution B: Apostrophe - 27

JUDICIAL ADDRESS TWO
Invention: Introduction to the Special Topics - 33
Arrangement: Refining the Exordium - 37
Elocution A: Terminating Sentences - 41
Elocution B: Citations - 43

JUDICIAL ADDRESS THREE
Invention: Justice - 49
Arrangement: Refining the Amplification -51
Elocution A: Compound Sentences - 54
Elocution B: Complex Sentences - 57

JUDICIAL ADDRESS FOUR
Invention: Evidence - 63
Arrangement: Refining the Refutation - 67
Elocution A: Anaphora - 70
Elocution B: Epistrophe - 73

JUDICIAL ADDRESS FIVE
Invention: Laws I - 79
Arrangement: Refining the Proof - 82
Elocution A: Synecdoche - 87
Elocution B: Sentence Amplification - 91

TABLE *of* CONTENTS

JUDICIAL ADDRESS SIX
Invention: Laws II - 99
Arrangement: Refining the Proof II - 103
Elocution A: Hyperbole - 107
Elocution B: Litotes - 111

JUDICIAL ADDRESS SEVEN
Invention Review - 116
Arrangement Review - 117
Elocution A: Erotema - 119
Elocution B: Hypophora - 121

APPENDICES
Tools of Invention - 126
Tools of Arrangement - 128
Tools of Elocution - 130
Sample Addresses - 133
Glossary - 150
Arrangement Templates - 153

COMPLETE PERSUASIVE ESSAY REVIEW

INVENTION WORKSHEET

Reviewing the Common Topics

Demonstrate how to use each of the five common topics by generating an example for each:

Definition

_____

_____

Comparison

_____

_____

Relation

_____

_____

Circumstance

_____

_____

Testimony

_____

_____

<u>Describe</u> how to use each of the five common topics:

Definition

_____

_____

Comparison

_____

_____

Relation

_____

_____

Circumstance

_____

_____

Testimony

_____

_____

Continue to use the common topics during Invention for all LTW II assignments.

ARRANGEMENT WORKSHEET

Reviewing the Outline

Complete the following to review the elements of Arrangement:

1. List each element of an outline.

_____

_____

_____

_____

_____

_____

2. Generate an outline for a complete persuasive essay.

Continue to use the elements of Arrangement in all LTW II assignments.

Complete Persuasive Essay: Outline

I. Introduction
   A. Exordium*
   B. Narratio
      1. Situation*
      2. Actions*
   C. Division
      1. Agreement*
      2. Disagreement
         a. Counter-thesis*
         b. Thesis*
   D. Distribution
      1. Thesis*
      2. Enumeration*
      3. Exposition
         a. Proof I*
         b. Proof II*
         c. Proof III*

II. Proof
   A. Proof I*
      1. Support 1*
      2. Support 2*
      3. Support 3*
   B. Proof II*
      1. Support 1*
      2. Support 2*
      3. Support 3*
   C. Proof III*
      1. Support 1*
      2. Support 2*
      3. Support 3*

III. Refutation
   A. Counter-thesis*
   B. Counter-proof I*
      1. Summary of support for counter-proof I*
      2. Inadequacy of counter-proof I*
   C. Counter-proof II*
      1. Summary of support for counter-proof II*
      2. Inadequacy of counter-proof II*
   D. Summary of Refutation*

IV. Conclusion
   A. Thesis*
   B. Summary of Proof
      1. Proof I*
      2. Proof II*
      3. Proof III*
   C. Amplification
      1. To whom it matters*
      2. Why it matters*

ELOCUTION WORKSHEET

Reviewing Schemes & Tropes

Complete the following to review the tools of Elocution:

1. Demonstrate your mastery of the tools of Elocution by generating an example of each of the following:

Parallelism

_____

_____

Antithesis

_____

_____

Simile

_____

_____

Alliteration

_____

_____

Metaphor

_____

_____

Assonance

_____

_____

Edited Verb

Vague Verb

Precise Verb

Write your complete persuasive essay and add each tool of Elocution.

JUDICIAL ADDRESS ONE

INVENTION WORKSHEET

Character Bias

There are two kinds of bias: for and against. In this exercise, you identify how a character is biased for or against the defendant, the action, and the victim. You will then add one additional bias.

Bias – The inclination to favor or oppose people, institutions, actions, things, ideas, or opinions. The word bias is Greek for "a leaning."

Defendant – The character accused of the action considered in the issue.

1. Express the issue in the form "whether X should have done Y."

_____

2. List four characters from the story.

A. _____

B. _____

C. _____

D. _____

3. Note whether the characters are inclined to favor or oppose the defendant and how they show their bias.

_____

_____

_____

_____

4. Note whether the characters are inclined to approve or disapprove of the action and how they show their bias.

_____

_____

_____

_____

5. Note whether the characters are inclined to favor or oppose the victim and how they show their bias.

_____

_____

_____

_____

6. Identify one more thing that each character manifests a bias for or against.

Character	Thing	Favors	Opposes	How it is shown
		☐	☐	
		☐	☐	
		☐	☐	
		☐	☐	

7. Move to ANI.

8. Review your I column and move appropriate items to A or N column.

20

ARRANGEMENT WORKSHEET

Refining the Narratio

Complete the following to develop a refined narratio. Your ANI may help identify causes.

1. Sort your ANI and identify the best proofs for the affirmative and negative. Choose your thesis based on which has the best proofs. If you choose the affirmative, you will want to defend the defendant against those who say he should not have done it. If you choose the negative, you are prosecuting him for having done it. The affirmative will want the audience to feel pity for the defendant. The negative will want the audience to feel indignation toward the defendant.

2. Describe the situation.

_____

_____

4. If you are defending the defendant (affirmative), identify an action, decision, or event that caused the situation and will elicit pity toward the defendant. If you are prosecuting the defendant (negative), identify an action, decision, or event that caused the situation and will elicit indignation toward the defendant.

_____

_____

3. What action, decision, or event led to this situation?

_____

_____

5. Identify the action, decision, or event that caused your answer to the previous question.

_____

_____

6. Identify additional causes as needed.

_____

_____

_____

_____

7. Rearrange the sequence above into a narratio outline in chronological order.

8. Add the narratio to your main outline.

    Narratio
      A. Cause 1**
      B. Cause 2**
      C. Cause 3**
      D. Situation**

** In previous outlines, you have left the name of the outline point (i.e., narratio) or replaced the name (i.e., Cause 1), but from now on with the double asterisk, you will include the name and your information in the outline point.

Complete Persuasive Essay: Outline

I. Introduction
    A. Exordium*
    B. Narratio
        1. Cause 1**
        2. Cause 2**
        3. Cause 3**
        4. Situation**
    C. Division
        1. Agreement*
        2. Disagreement
            a. Counter-thesis*
            b. Thesis*
    D. Distribution
        1. Thesis*
        2. Enumeration*
        3. Exposition
            a. Proof I*
            b. Proof II*
            c. Proof III*

II. Proof
    A. Proof I*
        1. Support 1*
        2. Support 2*
        3. Support 3*
    B. Proof II*
        1. Support 1*
        2. Support 2*
        3. Support 3*
    C. Proof III*
        1. Support 1*
        2. Support 2*
        3. Support 3*

III. Refutation
    A. Counter-thesis*
    B. Counter-proof I*
        1. Summary of support for counter-proof I*
        2. Inadequacy of counter-proof I*
    C. Counter-proof II*
        1. Summary of support for counter-proof II*
        2. Inadequacy of counter-proof II*
    D. Summary of Refutation*

IV. Conclusion
    A. Thesis*
    B. Summary of Proof
        1. Proof I*
        2. Proof II*
        3. Proof III*
    C. Amplification
        1. To Whom It Matters*
        2. Why It Matters*

ELOCUTION WORKSHEET A

Personification

Key Terms:

◇ **Personification**: A trope in which human characteristics are attributed to a non-human thing.

◇ **Trope**: A figure of speech that appeals to the mind or imagination.

◇ **Scheme**: A figure of speech that appeals to the senses.

Examples from Great Literature

Robert Louis Stevenson's "My Shadow"

One morning very early, before the sun was up,
I rose and found the shining dew on every buttercup;
But my lazy little shadow, like an errant sleepy-head,
Had stayed at home behind me and was fast asleep in bed.

Harper Lee's *To Kill a Mockingbird*

Nothing is more deadly than a deserted, waiting street.
The following week **the knot-hole yielded a tarnished medal.**

William Shakespeare's *Macbeth*, Act IV, Scene III

The sun's a thief, and **his great attraction robs the vast sea.**

Virgil's *Aeneid*

Then, swiftest of all evils, **Rumor runs
Straightway through Libya's mighty cities**—Rumor,
Whose life is speed, whose going gives her force.

J.A. Daly's *In Coventry*

My friends, the leaves, who used to entertain me
On summer afternoons with idle chatter,
Are dropping off in ways that shock and pain me.
I wonder what's the matter.

Steps to Writing Personification

1. Select a term to personify.
2. Define the term.
3. Identify human characteristics attributable to the term.
4. Write a sentence attributing a human characteristic to the term.

Practice

1. Personify a toy or tool you have used.

Term and definition:

_____

Human characteristic:

_____

Sentence:

_____

2. Personify something you can find in your imagination.

Term and definition:

_____

Human characteristic:

_____

Sentence:

_____

3. Personify something from a story.

Term and definition:

_____

Human characteristic:

_____

Sentence:

_____

4. Generate a personification, and add it to your essay.

ELOCUTION WORKSHEET B
Apostrophe

Key Terms:

◇ **Apostrophe:** A trope in which a writer speaks directly to a personified object, an absent person (including someone who is deceased), an abstraction, or oneself.

Examples from Great Literature

Alfred Lord Tennyson's "Break, Break, Break"

Break, break, break
On the cold gray stones, **O Sea!**

Bible, I Corinthians 15:55

O death, where is thy sting? **O grave,** where is thy victory?

William Shakespeare's *Macbeth*, V, Scene V

Out, Out, **brief candle**!

Maschwitz and Posford's "Goodnight, Vienna"

Goodnight, Vienna, you city of a million melodies...

William Shakespeare's *Julius Caesar*, Act III, Scene I

O pardon me, **thou bleeding piece of earth**,
That I am meek and gentle with these butchers!

Steps to Writing Personification

1. Identify something to address.
2. Identify a characteristic to emphasize.
3. List some things you might say to a human that shared the personified characteristic of that thing.
4. Choose one.
5. Write a sentence by speaking to the personified object.

Practice

1. Generate apostrophe by speaking to a tool or toy you use or have used.

Identify something to address:

_____

Identify a characteristic to emphasize:

_____

List some things you might say to a human that shared the personified characteristic of that thing:

_____

Choose one:

_____

Write a sentence by speaking to the personified object:

_____

2. Generate apostrophe by speaking to something in your imagination.

Identify something to address:

_____

Identify a characteristic to emphasize:

List some things you might say to a human that shared the personified characteristic of that thing:

Choose one:

Write a sentence by speaking to the personified object:

3. Generate apostrophe by speaking to something from a story.

Identify something to address:

Identify a characteristic to emphasize:

List some things you might say to a human that shared the personified characteristic of that thing:

Choose one:

Write a sentence by speaking to the personified object:

4. Add apostrophe to your essay.

JUDICIAL ADDRESS TWO

INVENTION WORKSHEET

Special Topics

Key Terms:

◇ **Special Topics:** Categories of questions used to gather information for a particular kind of address.

◇ **Justice:** A special topic that helps students discover whether an action is right or wrong, fair or unfair.

◇ **An Sit:** A special topic that helps students collect evidence to determine whether an act occurred and whether the defendant committed the act.

◇ **Quid Sit:** A special topic that helps students discover what happened and whether a law was violated.

◇ **Quale Sit:** A special topic that helps students discover why a defendant committed an act and whether the act is justifiable or excusable.

◇ **PDI:** A modification of the ANI table for the judicial address. It helps the student invent for judicial issues by collecting information for the prosecution and defense. P stands for prosecution, D for defense, and I for indeterminate.

I. Express the Issue in the form "whether X should be punished for Y."

2. Record your answers for the following questions in the PDI table.

Why might the action be unjust?
 - What about the action was appropriate (D)? What about the action was inappropriate (P)?
 - What about the action was right (D)? What about the action was wrong (P)?
 - What about the action was fair (D)? What about the action was unfair (P)?

An Sit. **Did the defendant do it?**
- What evidence indicates that the action happened?
- What evidence indicates that the defendant committed the action?

Quid Sit. **What happened?**
- What harms resulted (P)?
- What harms were prevented (D)?
- What rules were broken (P)?
- What rules were kept (D)?

Quale Sit. **Why did it happen?**
- What caused or motivated the defendant to commit the act (P/D)?
- What about the action is punishable (P)?
- For what reason might the action be excusable (D)?
- For what reason might the action be justifiable (D)?

Quale Sit. **What kind of person is the defendant?**
- List some of the defendant's virtues.
- List some of the defendant's vices.

PDI Table

P	D	I

ARRANGEMENT WORKSHEET

Refining the Exordium

Key Terms:

◇ **Bias to Blame:** The inclination of a judge to find fault in the victim or defendant.

◇ **Bias to Favor:** The inclination of a judge to excuse or praise the victim or defendant.

◇ **Bias to Approve:** The inclination of a judge to believe the action is generally appropriate.

◇ **Bias to Disapprove:** The inclination of a judge to believe the action is rarely appropriate.

◇ **Goodwill:** A favorable inclination or disposition.

◇ **Anecdote:** A short story about a real incident or person.

> **Nota Bene:** For the sake of the judicial address, students are free to create stories that are "real" to the fictional characters but imaginative to us.

◇ **Judicial Paradox:** A statement acknowledging that, while the victim or the defendant's action or character appears to confirm the judge's bias, the evidence will show the opposite.

◇ **Clarification:** A statement in which the student makes clear that while the judge expects him to argue X, he is actually going to argue Y.

◇ **Indirect Opening:** An Exordium that does not begin with the case itself.

> **Nota Bene:** *On rare occasions, speakers can proceed directly to the case itself, without an introduction. However, this approach is not taught in LTW I or II.*

◇ **Audience:** A character or group from the story other than the defendant, the victim, or a personal witness who will judge the case.

> **Nota Bene:** *LTW II uses the words "audience" and "judge" interchangeably.*

37

I. Write your thesis:

2. Select an audience by following the instructions below. Choose one inclined to disagree with your case:

List characters inclined to blame or favor the victim. Explain how they reveal their bias.

List characters inclined to blame or favor the defendant. Explain how they reveal their bias.

3. Having chosen a judge inclined to oppose your thesis, use either the prosecution or defense worksheet to generate an exordium appropriate to your thesis and audience:

Prosecution

A. If the judge is inclined to blame the victim, identify an **anecdote** that warns the judge of a time when showing mercy had negative consequences.

B. If the judge is inclined to favor the defendant, admit the **paradox** that the defendant's action or character appears to be innocent but isn't.

C. If the judge is inclined to approve of the action, **clarify** that while the judge thinks you are here to argue X, you are actually going to argue Y.

38

D. Add your exordium to the outline by selecting which of the three kinds of exordia you chose.

☐ Anecdote
☐ Paradox
☐ Clarification

E. Transition to narratio by telling when it happened (e.g., yesterday, last week). See sample essays for examples of transition to narratio.

F. Complete the outline

    I. Introduction
        A. Exordium* (i.e., anecdote, paradox, clarification)

Defense

A. If the judge is inclined to favor the victim, admit the paradox that the victim appears good but either isn't or that it doesn't matter in this case.

_____

_____

B. If the judge is inclined to blame the defendant, identify an anecdote that reminds the judge of a time when an innocent person was punished.

_____

_____

C. If the judge is inclined to disapprove of the action, clarify that while the judge thinks you are going to argue X, you are actually going to argue Y.

_____

_____

D. Add your exordium to the outline by selecting which of the three kinds of exordia you chose.

☐ Anecdote
☐ Paradox
☐ Clarification

E. Transition to narratio by telling when it happened (e.g., yesterday, last week). See sample essays for examples of transition to narratio.

F. Complete the outline

I. Introduction
A. Exordium* (i.e., snecdote, paradox, clarification)

ELOCUTION WORKSHEET A

Terminating Sentences

Key Terms:

◇ **Paragraph:** a sentence or group of sentences that develop a single idea.

◇ **Terminating Sentence:** The final sentence of a paragraph that terminates the paragraph's idea.

Steps to Writing Terminating Sentences

1. If the paragraph is long or complex, add a **summary sentence**.
2. If the paragraph leads you to draw a logical or practical conclusion, express that **conclusion**.
3. If the paragraph leads you to an insight, express that **insight**.
4. If the paragraph leads you to a moral application, add a **moral appeal.**
5. Add terminating sentences to the paragraphs in your case.

Practice

Generate terminating sentences for each paragraph in your case by following the instructions below.

1. If the paragraph is long or complex, add a summary sentence. To write your terminating sentence, you may imitate one of the following forms or generate your own.

    a. It is clear that _____

    b. In conclusion _____

    c. I have shown that _____

2. If the paragraph leads you to draw a logical or practical conclusion, express that conclusion. To write your terminating sentence, you may imitate one of the following forms or generate your own.

    a. It must be either _____ *or* _____

    b. At this rate _____

41

c. As a result _____

3. If the paragraph leads you to an insight, express that insight. To write your terminating sentence, you may imitate one of the following forms or generate your own.

    a. I now realize that _____

    b. It is better to X than Y _____

    c. This helped convince me that _____

4. If the paragraph leads you to make a moral application, add a moral appeal. To write your terminating sentence, you may imitate one of the following forms or generate your own.

    a. This is why we ought to _____

    b. It is only right that _____

    c. A just person would _____

5. Add a terminating sentence to each paragraph in your case. Beginning with Judicial Address Three, you will add a terminating sentence to your outline by identifying its kind.

ELOCUTION WORKSHEET B

Citations

Complete the Citations Table following the steps below:

1. With your outline beside you, identify those proofs that need additional support by checking box 'C' for Citation Needed or 'N' for Not Needed. Use the following questions to help make that determination.

a. Argumentative: Would support from the text strengthen my argument?

b. Interpretive: Would my interpretation benefit from additional support?

c. Informative: Would additional information help support or explain my argument?

2. If you answer yes to any of the above questions, mark the argument as Citation Needed 'C' and choose one of the following citations:

a. Text: Add a quotation or paraphrase from the story text, providing the page or line number.

b. Authority: Add a statement from another source that supports your interpretation specifically (e.g., a commentary or article) or generally (e.g., Scripture, U.S. Constitution, maxims, ethical writings, etc.), providing the source name and page number, line number, or verse where it can be found.

c. Reference: Add a definition or additional information that strengthens the argument, providing the information and the source.

Add the information to your address, and cite it. Include the citation in parentheses at the end of the sentence, or follow an approved style guide. Add quotations to the argument (using quotation marks), and including a citation at the end of the sentence in parentheses.

Citations Table

Case	C:	N:	Citation
Argument 1			
1.			
2.			
3.			
Argument 2			
1.			
2.			
3.			
Argument 3			
1.			
2.			
3.			

Additional Elocution Practice

Level I Schemes: parallelism, antithesis, alliteration, assonance
Level I Tropes: simile, metaphor
Level II Tropes: personification, apostrophe

On a separate sheet of paper:

Write an example of parallelism.

Write an example of antithesis.

Write an example of alliteration.

Write an example of assonance.

Write an example of simile.

Write an example of metaphor.

Write an example of personification.

Write an example of apostrophe.

Add at least two of the schemes and/or tropes you reviewed to your address. Also add the new tools of elocution.

JUDICIAL ADDRESS THREE

INVENTION WORKSHEET

Special Topics: Justice

Use the worksheet below to practice gathering information to determine whether an action is just. You will use the same four steps twice—once imagining yourself as the prosecutor and once imagining yourself as the defense.

All information will be recorded in your PDI.

Key Terms:

◇ **Justice:** The quality of an action that treats persons, things, or situations appropriately.

◇ **Right:** The quality of an action being appropriate to a situation.

◇ **Fair:** The quality of an action being an appropriate response to a person or thing.

◇ **Appropriate:** The quality of being suitable or proper to the circumstances.

◇ **Rule:** An expressed expectation or requirement that a person behave a certain way; it can be either written or unwritten, spoken or unspoken.

Practice

Express your issue in the form "Whether X should be punished for Y."

Assume the role of prosecutor and gather information for the P column, using the common and special topics.

Gather additional information for the P column using the special topic of justice by answering the following questions.

- In what way was the action inappropriate (if any)?

49

- In what way was the action wrong (if any)?

- In what way was the action unfair (if any)?

- What rules were broken?

- If any were, who made the rules?

Sort the P column.

List the three best arguments.

_____

_____

_____

Assume the role of defense and gather information for the D column, using the common and special topics.

Gather additional information for the D column using the special topic of justice by answering the following questions.

- In what way was the action appropriate (if any)?

- In what way was the action right (if any)?

- In what way was the action fair (if any)?

- What rules were kept?

- If any were, who made those rules?

Sort the D column.

List the three best arguments.

_____

_____

_____

ARRANGEMENT WORKSHEET

Refining the Amplification

Key Terms:

◇ **Appeal to Emotion:** A way of communicating that elicits an emotion from the audience (i.e., hope or fear, anger or pity).

Practice

Choose a thesis:

Compare the prosecution's case with the defense's case, determine which is the stronger case, and decide whether to prosecute or defend.

_____

_____

Identify your audience.

_____

Elicit a response:

Identify people, things, or institutions that would be affected by the judge's decision.

_____

_____

Circle three about which the judge cares.

Choose one that would be significantly affected by the judge's decision.

_____

51

To elicit fear: If the audience judges the case as it is inclined, how will the person, thing, or institution be harmed?

_____

_____

To elicit hope: If the audience judges the case against its inclination, how will the person, thing, or institution be benefitted?

_____

_____

Choose an amplification:

Choose which amplification is most appropriate based on whether you are trying to elicit hope or fear from the judge.

Add to the outline:

I. Amplification: Appeal to fear or to hope?
      A. What does the judge care about?
      B. How will it be affected?

Judicial Address Three: Outline

I. **Introduction**
   A. Kind of Exordium*
   B. Narratio
      1. Cause 1**
      2. Cause 2**
      3. Cause 3**
      4. Situation**
   C. Division
      1. Agreement*
      2. Disagreement
         a. Counter-Thesis*
         b. Thesis*
   D. Distribution
      1. Thesis*
      2. Enumeration*
      3. Exposition
         a. Argument I*
         b. Argument II*
         c. Argument III*

II. **Case**
   A. Argument I*
      1. Support 1*
      2. Support 2*
      3. Support 3*
      4. Kind of Terminating Sentence*
   B. Argument II*
      1. Support 1*
      2. Support 2*
      3. Support 3*
      4. Kind of Terminating Sentence*
   C. Argument III*
      1. Support 1*
      2. Support 2*
      3. Support 3*
      4. Kind of Terminating Sentence*

III. **Refutation**
   A. Counter-Thesis*
   B. Counter-Argument I*
      1. Summary of support for Counter-Argument I*
      2. Inadequacy of Counter-Argument I*
   C. Counter-Argument II*
      1. Summary of support for Counter-Argument II*
      2. Inadequacy of Counter-Argument II*
   D. Summary of Refutation*

IV. **Conclusion**
   A. Thesis*
   B. Summary of Case
      1. Argument I*
      2. Argument II*
      3. Argument III*
   C. Amplification
      1. What does the judge care about?*
      2. How will it be affected?*

ELOCUTION WORKSHEET A

Compound Sentences

Key Terms:

◇ **Clause:** An expression of words that contains both a subject and a predicate; it can stand alone as a complete sentence or be joined to other words, phrases, or clauses as part of a larger sentence.

◇ **Coordinating Clause:** A clause joined to another clause or sentence by use of a comma and a coordinating conjunction (e.g., and, or, but, yet, nor, for, so) or a semicolon, in order to create a compound sentence.

◇ **Coordinating Conjunction**: A conjunction that joins two or more clauses.

◇ **Simple Sentence:** A sentence that consists of one independent clause.

◇ **Compound Sentence:** A sentence that consists of two or more independent clauses, joined by a coordinating conjunction and a comma or by a semicolon.

Review

List the parts of speech:

_____

_____

Define clause:

_____

_____

List the coordinating conjunctions:

_____

_____

Examples from Great Literature

Flannery O'Connor's "The Crop"

She could usually think best sitting in front of her typewriter, but this would do for the time being.

Harper Lee's *To Kill a Mockingbird*

What Jem called the Dewey Decimal System was school wide by the end of my first year, so I had no chance to compare it with other teaching techniques.

Proverbs 16:4

He who seeks the Lord will find knowledge with righteousness, and those who seek Him rightly will find peace.

Grimm Brothers' "The Raven"

She flew into a dark wood, and her parents did not know what had become of her.

Daniel Defoe's *Robinson Crusoe*

We made signs of thanks to them, for we had nothing to make them amends.

Steps

1. Find or create two simple sentences.

2. Join the two sentences together with a comma followed by the appropriate conjunction or by using a semi-colon in place of both. Coordinating conjunctions include "and," "or," "but," "yet," "nor," "so," and "for."

3. Write the result as a compound sentence.

Practice

1. Generate a compound sentence using two simple sentences from your address:

_____

_____

2. Generate compound sentences from the following clauses:

My house is a mess.	*The dog is loose in the neighborhood.*	*Cats are cool.*
The girl is brave.	*The boy loves math.*	*She is eating.*
Her bedroom is pink.	*He works at the gas station.*	*It smells nice.*

_____

_____

_____

_____

_____

3. Generate a compound sentence from simple sentences you create:

_____

_____

_____

_____

_____

4. Add compound sentences to your address.

ELOCUTION WORKSHEET B

Complex Sentences

Key Terms:

◇ **Subordinating Conjunction**: A conjunction that marks a clause as the subordinate clause when joined to another clause

◇ **Subordinate Clause:** A dependent clause joined to an independent clause by means of a subordinating conjunction (after, although, as, because, before, even, whereas, since, unless, etc.) in order to create a complex sentence

◇ **Complex Sentence**: A sentence with an independent clause and one or more subordinate (dependent) clauses

Review

Describe how a dependent clause is different from an independent clause:

_____

_____

List subordinating conjunctions:

_____

_____

Examples from Great Literature

Harper Lee's *To Kill a Mockingbird*

When he was nearly thirteen, my brother Jem got his arm badly broken at the elbow.

Isaiah 53:7

Although he was ill-treated, He opened not His mouth.

Andrew Lang's *The Lilac Fairy Book*, "The Stones of Plouhinec"

As he was passing the long line of stones, he saw Bernèz working with a chisel on the tallest of them all.

Aesop's "The Milk-woman and Her Pail"

A farmer's daughter was carrying her pail of milk from the field to the farm-house, when she fell a-musing.

Flannery O'Connor's "Good Country People"

"She's got to eat," Mrs. Hopewell muttered, sipping her coffee, while she watched Joy's back at the stove.

Steps

1. Find or create two simple sentences.

2. Choose a subordinating conjunction. (Subordinating conjunctions include after, although, as, because, before, even, whereas, since, unless...).

3. Add the subordinating conjunction to the beginning of one of the two simple sentences, thus turning it into a subordinate clause.

4. Combine the two sentences. When the subordinate clause comes first, insert a comma between the clauses. When the subordinate clause comes second, do not insert a comma.

Practice

1. Generate a complex sentence using two simple sentences from your address:

_____

_____

2. Generate complex sentences from the following clauses:

Julia asked for a cup of hot chocolate.	*He works at the gas station.*
That bluff has been called.	*I thought she was safe.*
The dog is loose in the neighborhood.	*We musn't leave.*
Their voices were straining to be heard.	*Someone sent them to Celia.*

_____

_____

_____

_____

_____

3. Generate a complex sentence from simple sentences you create:

_____

_____

_____

_____

_____

4. Add complex sentences to your address.

Additional Elocution Practice

Level I Schemes: parallelism, antithesis, alliteration, assonance
Level I Tropes: simile, metaphor
Level II Schemes: compound sentences
Level II Tropes: personification, apostrophe

On a separate sheet of paper write . . .

1. An example of parallelism

2. An example of antithesis

3. An example of alliteration

4. An example of assonance

5. An example of simile

6. An example of metaphor

7. An example of personification

8. An example of apostrophe

9. An example of a compound sentence

10. An example of a complex sentence

11. An example of anaphora

12. An example of epistrophe

Add at least two of the reviewed schemes and/or tropes to your address. Also add at least one compound and one complex sentence (you may do so by combining sentences already written).

JUDICIAL ADDRESS FOUR

INVENTION WORKSHEET

Special Topics: Evidence

Key Terms:

◇ **An Sit:** A special topic of invention for judicial issues, used to determine if there is enough evidence to prove the defendant committed the act.

◇ **An Sit Issue:** An issue expressed in the form "Whether X did Y."

◇ **Evidence:** Any information used by the prosecution or defense in a judicial address to prove the defendant committed or didn't commit the act—it includes <u>physical</u> and <u>personal</u> evidence.

◇ **Physical Evidence:** The facts, data, and physical things (forensics) that indicate the guilt or innocence of the defendant.

◇ **Personal Evidence**

> • **Eyewitness:** Anyone who witnessed the act or the circumstances in which it occurred, or who can provide an alibi (ie., testify to the defendant's absence: "alibi" is Latin for "elsewhere").

> • **Expert Witness:** A person with the authority to interpret the material evidence and determine whether it supports the case for the prosecution or for the defense's case.

> • **Character Witness:** A person who can testify to the quality of another person's character (i.e., virtues and/or vices).

◇ **Relevant:** An attribute of evidence that pertains to or sustains the argument to which it is applied.

◇ **Reliable:** An attribute of evidence that is what the prosecution or defense claims it to be.

◇ **Credible:** An attribute of testimony that is what the witness claims it to be.

63

Practice

1. Express the issue (be sure to use a legally neutral verb to describe the action) in the form "Whether X did Y."

2. Evaluate the case for the prosecution.

Physical Evidence Table

List physical evidence	Who reported the evidence? (the witness)	What is the witness' bias?	Who interpreted evidence?	What is their interpretation?	What is their bias?	How is the evidence relevant to the case?

Personal Evidence Table

List testimonials	Who reported the testimony?	How might it be challenged?	What is the eyewitness' bias?	How is the testimony relevant to the case?

3. Transfer the information to the P column of the PDI.

4. Sort the P column.

5. Evaluate the case for the defense.

Present the case for the prosecution	Look for weakness in the case for the prosecution		
List prosecution's arguments or their key evidence	Is evidence factually correct?	Is there any counter-evidence?	Is the Conclusion (the Case for the Prosecution) Logically Necessary? (Explain)
1.			
2.			
3.			

Use the questions from the prosecution tables to evaluate counter-evidence.

In the row that contains the prosecution's evidence, evaluate each individual evidence to determine whether it shows that the defendant probably or necessarily committed the act. In the box in the bottom row, evaluate all three of the prosecution's arguments/evidence together to determine whether the whole case proves (i.e., shows to be logically necessary or probable) that the defendant committed the act.

6. Transfer information to D column of the PDI.

ARRANGEMENT WORKSHEET

Refining the Refutation

Key Terms:

◇ **Refining the Refuation:** The prosecution refutes the defense's case. Because the defense's case is already a refutation of the prosecution's case, he will write a rebuttal, attempting to rebuild his case after the prosecution's refutation.

◇ **Refutation:** A response to an opposing case that shows it to be false.

Steps to Refine the Refutation

1. List the prosecution's three arguments.

2. List the defense's three arguments.

3. Generate the prosecution's refutation of the defense's arguments. Use this as your refutation if you are the prosecutor.

    a. Identify two summary arguments for the defense.

    b. Explain why each is inadequate.

4. Rebuild the defense's case.

    a. Move the prosecution's two arguments for inadequacy from 3B to the first and third boxes under the defense's refutation.

    b. Explain why the defense arguments actually are adequate.

67

Practice Refutation

	Prosecution's case	Defense's case
Argument 1		
Argument 2		
Argument 3		
	Prosecution's refutation	**Defense's refutation**
Defense 1		
Why inadequate?		
Defense 2		
Why inadequate?		
Prosecution's argument for inadequacy 1		
Why is D1 adequate?		
Prosecution's argument for inadequacy 2		
Why is D2 adequate?		

Add to outline.

JUDICIAL ADDRESS FOUR: ARRANGEMENT TEMPLATE

I. **Introduction**
   A. Kind of Exordium*
   B. Narratio
      1. Cause 1**
      2. Cause 2**
      3. Cause 3**
      4. Situation**
   C. Division
      1. Agreement*
      2. Disagreement
         a. Counter-Thesis*
         b. Thesis*
   D. Distribution
      1. Thesis*
      2. Enumeration*
      3. Exposition
         a. Argument I*
         b. Argument II*
         c. Argument III*

II. **Case**
   A. Argument I*
      1. Support 1*
      2. Support 2*
      3. Support 3*
      4. Kind of Terminating Sentence*
   B. Argument II*
      1. Support 1*
      2. Support 2*
      3. Support 3*
      4. Kind of Terminating Sentence*
   C. Argument III*
      1. Support 1*
      2. Support 2*
      3. Support 3*
      4. Kind of Terminating Sentence*

III. **Refutation**
   A. Counter-Thesis*
   B. Counter-Argument I*
      1. Summary of support for Counter-Argument I*
      2. Inadequacy of Counter-Argument I*
   C. Counter-Argument II*
      1. Summary of support for Counter-Argument II*
      2. Inadequacy of Counter-Argument II*
   D. Summary of Refutation*

IV. **Conclusion**
   A. Thesis*
   B. Summary of Case
      1. Argument I*
      2. Argument II*
      3. Argument III*
   C. Amplification
      1. What does the judge care about?*
      2. How will it be affected?*

ELOCUTION WORKSHEET A

Anaphora

Key Terms:

◇ **Anaphora:** A scheme in which a word, phrase, or clause is repeated at the beginning of successive phrases, clauses, and sentences.

Examples from Great Literature

Bible, Psalm 29:1

> **Bring to the Lord,** O you sons of God,
> **Bring to the Lord** the sons of rams;
> **Bring to the Lord** glory and honor.

Charles Dickens' *A Tale of Two Cities*

> **It was the** best of times, **it was the** worst of times,
> **it was the** age of wisdom, **it was the** age of foolishness . . .

William Shakespeare's *The Life and Death of King John*, Act II, Scene I

> **Mad** world! **Mad** kings! **Mad** composition!

Winston Churchill's "Speech to the House of Commons on June 4, 1940"

> **We shall fight** on the beaches, **we shall fight** on the landing grounds, **we shall fight** in the fields and in the streets, **we shall fight** in the hills; we shall never surrender...

Edmund Burke's "A Letter to a Noble Lord"

> **It is** a luxury, **it is** a privilege, **it is** an indulgence for those who are at their ease.

Steps

1. Select an idea, action, or quality to emphasize.

2. List three things true of that idea, action, or quality.

3. Write three phrases, clauses, or sentences that all begin with (repeat) the idea being emphasized.

Practice

1. Write anaphora for a tool or toy you use or have used:

Three things that are true

_____

_____

_____

Three phrases

_____

_____

_____

2. Write anaphora for something in your imagination:

Three things that are true

_____

_____

_____

Three phrases

3. Write anaphora for something from a story:

Three things that are true

Three phrases

4. Add anaphora to your address.

ELOCUTION WORKSHEET B
Epistrophe

Key Terms:

◇ **Epistrophe:** A scheme in which a word, phrase, or clause is repeated at the end of successive phrases, clauses, or sentences.

Examples from Great Literature

Abraham Lincoln's "Gettysburg Address"

Government of **the people,** by **the people,** for **the people.**

Bible, 1 Corinthians 13:11

When I was **a child,** I spoke as **a child,** I understood as **a child,** I thought as **a child.**

Malcolm X's *Message to the Grassroots*

As long as the white man sent you to Korea, **you bled.** He sent you to Germany, **you bled.** He sent you to the South Pacific to fight the Japanese, **you bled.**

William Shakespeare's *Merchant of Venice*, Act III, Scene III

I'll have **my bond!**
Speak not against **my bond!**
I have sworn an oath
that I will have **my bond.**

Ovid

If you **the sea held,** I would follow you, my wife,
Until me also **the sea held.**

Steps

1. Select an idea, action, or quality to emphasize.

2. List three things true of that idea, word, or phrase.

3. Write three phrases, clauses, or sentences that end with (repeat) the idea being emphasized.

Practice

1. Write epistrophe for a tool or toy you use or have used:

Three things that are true

_____

_____

_____

Three phrases

_____

_____

_____

2. Write epistrophe for a tool or toy you use or have used:

Three things that are true

_____

_____

_____

Three phrases

_____

_____

_____

3. Write epistrophe for something from a story:

Three things that are true

_____

_____

_____

Three phrases

_____

_____

_____

4. Add epistrophe to your address.

Additional Elocution Practice

Level I Schemes: parallelism, antithesis, alliteration, assonance
Level I Tropes: simile, metaphor
Level II Schemes: compound sentence, complex sentence
Level II Tropes: personification, apostrophe, anaphora, epistrophe

On a separate sheet of paper write:

1. An example of parallelism

2. An example of antithesis

3. An example of alliteration

4. An example of assonance

5. An example of simile

6. An example of metaphor

7. An example of personification

8. An example of apostrophe

9. An example of a compound sentence

10. An example of a complex sentence

Add at least two of the schemes and/or tropes you reviewed to your address.

Also add epistrophe and apostrophe.

JUDICIAL ADDRESS FIVE

INVENTION WORKSHEET

Laws I

Key Terms:

◇ **Quid Sit:** A special topic that helps students discover what happened and whether a law was violated.

◇ **Quale Sit:** A special topic that helps students discover why a defendant committed an act and whether the act was justifiable or excusable.

Practice

Express the issue (be sure to use a legally neutral verb to describe the action) in the form "Whether X did Y."

ASSUME THE ROLE OF PROSECUTOR

Record your information in the P or I columns or on separate paper if you find it helpful or necessary. Use the common topics, justice, and an sit to generate information for the case for prosecution. Imitate the tables and questions from earlier lessons as needed.

1. *Quid Sit*: Determine the laws broken.

- What natural laws were broken?
- What customary laws were broken?
- In what way did the action break the law?

2. *Quale Sit*: Determine the causes and motives of the defendant's action.

- Cause: What forces moved the defendant to act?
- Cause: Did the defendant break the law willingly?
- Motive: Why did the defendant commit the act (what did he hope for or fear)?

3. Sort the P column.

4. Conduct a friendly evaluation of the case for the prosecution to determine three argu-

79

ments that convincingly argue that the defendant broke a law without a sufficient excuse. List evidence, state the law broken, and show that the action was inexcusable.

Because the prosecution must always answer three questions—did he do it, what law did he break, and is it excusable—the three arguments for this address include two that present evidence to show the defendant acted as charged and one that shows that the action broke a law without a sufficient excuse.

ASSUME THE ROLE OF DEFENSE
Conduct a hostile evaluation of the case for the prosecution, asking the following questions. Record your answers under D or I on the PDI table or on the next page if you find it helpful or necessary.

1. Evaluate the ***an sit*** arguments.

- Is the evidence factually correct? Explain.
- Is there counter-evidence (e.g., an alibi)? Describe.
- If the combined evidence is not convincing, explain how the conclusion is not logically necessary.

2. Evaluate the ***quid sit*** arguments.

- Is there some way the specific action kept the law?
- Do you acknowledge that the defendant broke the law?

3. Evaluate the ***quale sit*** arguments.

- What caused the defendant to act? Was the act excusable?
- What was the defendant's motive (what did he hope for or fear?)? Was the act justifiable?

4. Sort the D Column.

5. Identify three arguments that convincingly demonstrate that the defendant did not do what he is accused of (*an sit*), did not break a law (*quid sit*), or either had an excuse or was justified in his action (*quale sit*).

"D" Notes:

ARRANGEMENT WORKSHEET

Refining the Case & the Refutation

Part One: Generate the Outline

1. Express your thesis in the form "Whether X should be punished for Y."

2. Generate your outline by completing the table below.

Prosecution	Defense
Evidence I:	Argument I:
I.	I.
2.	2.
3.	3.
Evidence 2	Argument 2:
I.	I.
2.	2.
3.	3.
Law Broken & Cause/Motive:	Argument 3:
I.	I.
2.	2.
3.	3.

Part 2: Generate the Refutation for the Prosecution

1. List the prosecution and defense arguments in the chart in part 3.

2. Refute the case for the defense. Record answers in the chart in part 3.

Choose whether the case for the defense is arguing that:

☐ *There is not enough evidence to prove the defendant acted* (an sit).

☐ *Though the defendant acted, he did not break a law* (quid sit).

☐ *Though the defendant broke a law, he was excused or justified* (quale sit).

Part 3: Generate the Refutation for the Defense

1. Summarize the case for the defense.

2. Explain why the prosecution fails to refute the case for the defense.

	Prosecution's Case	Defense's Case
Argument I:		
Argument 2:		
Argument 3:		
	Prosecution's Refutation	**Defense's Refutation**
Defense I:		
Why inadequate?		
Defense 2:		
Why inadequate?		
Prosecution's argument for inadequacy I		
Why is DI adequate?		
Prosecution's argument for inadequacy 2		
Why is D2 adequate?		

Add the appropriate refutation to your outline.

JUDICIAL ADDRESS FIVE: ARRANGEMENT TEMPLATE

I. **Introduction**
   A. Kind of Exordium*
   B. Narratio
      1. Cause 1**
      2. Cause 2**
      3. Cause 3**
      4. Situation**
   C. Division
      1. Agreement*
      2. Disagreement
         a. Counter-Thesis*
         b. Thesis*
   D. Distribution
      1. Thesis*
      2. Enumeration*
      3. Exposition
         a. Argument I*
         b. Argument II*
         c. Argument III*
II. **Case**
   A. Argument I*
      1. Support 1*
      2. Support 2*
      3. Support 3*
      4. Kind of Terminating Sentence*
   B. Argument II*
      1. Support 1*
      2. Support 2*
      3. Support 3*
      4. Kind of Terminating Sentence*
   C. Argument III*
      1. Support 1*
      2. Support 2*
      3. Support 3*
      4. Kind of Terminating Sentence*
III. **Refutation**
   A. Counter-Thesis*
   B. Counter-Argument I*
      1. Summary of support for Counter-Argument I*
      2. Inadequacy of Counter-Argument I*
   C. Counter-Argument II*
      1. Summary of support for Counter-Argument II*
      2. Inadequacy of Counter-Argument II*
   D. Summary of Refutation*
IV. **Conclusion**
   A. Thesis*
   B. Summary of Case
      1. Argument I*
      2. Argument II*
      3. Argument III*
   C. Amplification
      1. What does the judge care about?*
      2. How will it be affected?*

ELOCUTION WORKSHEET A

Synecdoche

Key Terms:

◇ **Synecdoche:** A trope in which a part of a thing is used to name or represent the whole.

Examples from Great Literature

William Shakespeare's *Macbeth*, Act V, Scene III

Take **thy face** hence.

Rudyard Kipling, *The Jungle Book*

"Oh you, stupid **tuft of feathers!**" said Rikki-tikki, angrily. "Is this the time to sing?"

William Shakespeare's *The Tempest*, Act III, Scene I

Miranda: My husband then?
Ferdinand: Ay, with a heart as willing
As bondage e'er of freedom: here's **my hand**

Steps to Write Synecdoche

1. Choose a term.

2. List its parts or members (physical and non-physical).

3. Choose a part or member that effectively represents the term.

4. Substitute the part for the term in the sentence.

Practice

1. Write synecdoche for a tool or toy you use or have used:

Object

_____

Parts or members

_____

_____

Select one to substitute for the whole

_____

_____

_____

2. Write synecdoche for something you can find in your imagination:

Object

_____

Parts or members

_____

_____

Select one to substitute for the whole:

_____

_____

_____

3. Write synecdoche for something from a story:

Object

_____

Parts or members

_____

_____

Select one to substitute for the whole:

_____

_____

_____

4. Add synecdoche to your address.

ELOCUTION WORKSHEET B

Sentence Amplification

Key Terms:

◊ **Ampification:** The act of expanding (amplifying) an idea by thinking about it from various angles.

◊ **Clause:** An expression that contains both a subject and a predicate; it can stand alone as a complete sentence or be joined to other clauses as part of a larger sentence. (Some grammarians argue that if it is a sentence, it is not a clause; others argue that a simple sentence is a clause. Students should feel free to regard a sentence as a clause.)

◊ **Coordinating Conjunction:** A conjunction that joins two or more words, clauses, or sentences.

◊ **Subordinating Conjunction:** A conjunction that joins a subordinate clause to an independent clause.

◊ **Subordinate Clause:** A dependent clause joined to an independent clause by means of a subordinating conjunction ("after," "although," "as," "because," "before," "even," "whereas," "since," "unless," etc.) in order to create a complex sentence.

◊ **Participle:** A word formed by tranfsorming a verb into an adjective (*thundering denunciation* and *chosen path*) or noun (*wonderful plan* and *wrong doing*).

◊ **Relative Pronoun:** A word that stands in the place of a noun and can be used to connect a phrase or clause to a noun or pronoun ("who," "which," "that," etc.) (*Let us shun everything that is offensive.*)

Examples from Great Literature

Examples from Judicial Address Three Elocution can and should also be used.

Pedraic Colum's *The Golden Fleece*

She told Medea that one day she would meet a woman **who** knew nothing about enchantments.

Jonathan Swift's *A Tale of a Tub*

Having, therefore, so narrowly **passed** through the intricate difficulty, the reader will, I am sure, agree with me on the conclusion . . .

Virgil's *Aeneid*

Orpheus accompanies, **plucking** his seven notes
Now with his fingers, now with his ivory quill

Virgil's *Aeneid*

But at Aeneas' side, the Sybil spoke, **warning** him briefly.

Virgil's *Aeneid*

And **who** is that one, Father,
Walking beside the captain as he comes?

Steps to Amplifying Sentences

Generate a Compound Sentence

1. Begin with a base clause.

2. Add a coordinating conjunction. Remember, the comma precedes the conjunction in a compound sentence.

3. Add a coordinate clause using one of the following modes:

- Add something (and, but also)
- Show contrast (but, however)
- Show cause and effect (so, therefore)
- Present a choice (or)

Generate a Complex Sentence

1. Begin with a base clause.

2. Add a dependent clause using one or more of the following means (to generate ideas you might ask what was the subject or object of the base clause doing, being, having, or experiencing):

- Add a subordinate clause before the clause.
- Add a subordinating conjunction to the base clause and follow it with a

dependent clause.
• Add a dependent clause using a relative pronoun (who, which, that). This dependant clause can go before, in the middle of, or after the base clause.
• Add a dependent clause using a present or past participle. This dependent clause can go before, in the middle, or after the base clause.

Amplify with a Scheme

1. Begin with a base clause.

2. Add a conjunction.

3. Generate a clause using a scheme (any scheme can be used once the students know them).

TIP

Remember: If no conjunction is used and the clauses are independent clauses, a semicolon is required to separate them.

Practice

_____

1. Amplify with a compound sentence.

The girl is allergic to peanut butter, and

_____

Pluto was a planet, however

_____

It is raining, therefore

_____

He likes running in races, or

_____

2. Amplify with a complex sentence. Add at least one relative pronoun and one participle:

The dog smells funny although
_____

Cats are better than dogs because

_____

Since the earth is round,

_____

Unless the Lord builds the house,

_____

3. Amplify with a scheme:

Telemachus sailed the wine-dark sea (use anaphora)

_____

A ghost appeared to Hamlet (use anaphora)

_____

Socrates drank the hemlock (use epistrophe)

_____

The boy wants a hot dog (use epistrophe)

_____

4. Add amplified sentences to your address.

Additional Elocution Practice

Level I Schemes: parallelism, antithesis, alliteration, assonance
Level I Tropes: simile, metaphor
Level II Schemes: compound sentence, complex sentence, amplified sentence
Level II Tropes: personification, apostrophe, anaphora, epistrophe

On a separate sheet of paper write . . .

1. An example of parallelism

2. An example of antithesis

3. An example of alliteration

4. An example of assonance

5. An example of simile

6. An example of metaphor

7. An example of personification

8. An example of apostrophe

9. An example of a compound sentence

10. An example of a complex sentence

11. An example of anaphora

12. An example of epistrophe

13. An example of synecdoche

14. An example of an amplified sentence

Add at least two of the schemes and/or tropes you reviewed to your address.

Also add synecdoche and sentence amplification.

95

JUDICIAL ADDRESS SIX

INVENTION WORKSHEET

Laws: Part II

Key Terms:

◇ **Cause**: A force that moves or influences a person to act or react in a given manner. The manner in which a person commits an act: intentionally, accidentally, by compulsion, or with premeditation. In some cases it excuses the act, in other cases it calls for punishment.

◇ **Motive:** The intentional cause; the hopes or fears that lead a person to act in a given way. The reason a person commits an act; in some cases it justifies the

Practice

Express the issue (be sure to use a legally neutral verb to describe the action) in the form of "Whether X did Y."

ASSUME THE ROLE OF PROSECUTOR
Record your information in the P Column. Use the common topics, justice, and an sit to generate information for the case for prosecution. Use tables and questions from earlier lessons as needed.

1. Use the **stasis topics** to further develop the case for the prosecution.

   A. *Quid Sit*: Determine the laws broken.

   • What **Natural Laws** were broken, if any (Refer to the tables for more details and examples of each of these laws)?

      - Laws of reverance: Laws that apply to those you are dependent on

      - Laws of equity: Laws that apply to peers

      - Laws of Benevolence: Laws that apply to your dependents

   • What **customary laws** were broken, if any (Refer to the tables for more details and examples of each of these laws)?

      - Laws of covenant: Contracts between two or more people

- Laws of statute: Legislation from the government

- Laws of Tradition: Customs handed down informally from earlier generations

B. _Quale Sit_: Determine the causes and motives of the defendant's action.

• Cause: Did the defendant know the law he was breaking?

• Cause: Did the defendant break the law willingly?

- Did he break the law by chance? Explain how. Is that a sufficient excuse? Explain.

- Did he break the law by compulsion? Explain how. Is that a sufficient excuse? Explain.

- Did he break the law because of habits? Explain how. Is that a sufficient excuse? Explain.

- Did he break the law by premeditation? Explain how. Is that a sufficient excuse? Explain.

• Motive: Why did the defendant commit the act? Explain what he was trying to gain or avoid, such as profit or loss, revenge or reward, punishment or pleasure.

• Motive: Is the defendant's action justified?

- Is there a higher law that justifies the defendant's action? (See the table "Hierarchy of Laws" for ideas).

2. Sort the P column.

3. Conduct a friendly evaluation of the case for the prosecution (the P column) to determine three arguments that convincingly argue that the defendant broke a law without a sufficient excuse. Choose three arguments that answer the questions:

• Did he do it?

• Did it break a law?

• Why isn't the action excusable or justifiable?

ASSUME THE ROLE OF THE DEFENSE
Conduct a hostile evaluation of the case for the prosecution, asking the following questions. Record your answers under D on the PDI table.

Evaluate the **_an sit_** arguments

• Is the evidence factually correct? Explain.

• Is there counter-evidence (e.g., an alibi)? Describe.

• If the combined evidence is not convincing, explain how the conclusion is not logically necessary.

2. Evaluate the *Quid Sit* arguments.

   • In what way did the action keep the law?

   • Do you acknowledge that the defendant broke the law?

3. Evaluate the *Quale Sit* arguments.

   • What caused the defendant to act? Is the act excusable?

   • What was the defendant's motive (what did he hope for or fear)?

   • What higher law justified the defendant's action? Explain. See the "Hierarhy of Laws" table on the next page for ideas.

4. Sort the D Column.

5. Identify three arguments that convincingly demonstrate that the defendant is not guilty of breaking the law, was keeping a higher law, or was justified in his action.

HIERARCHY OF LAWS TABLE

A defendant sometimes appeals to one law to justify breaking another. This is called the appeal to higher law.

Below are two different hierarchies of law: the Roman Table and the Hebrew Table. The Roman Table represents the hierarchical order that seems implied by Cicero. The Hebrew Table represents the hierarchical order that seems implied by the Hebrew tradition. Both the defense and the prosecution may find these tables useful to reflect on whether the defendant's action can be justified.

ROMAN TABLE

Laws of Nature

> Religion - Honor to God
> Duty - Honor to homeland and family
> Gratitude – Honor to giver, patron
> Vengeance – Honor for victim
> Reverence – Honor to a superior or authority
> Truth – Honor to facts

Laws of Custom

> Law of Covenant – agreement between persons
> Law of Equity – fairness to others
> Law of Statute – written law or understood customs

HEBREW TABLE

Law of Reverence

> To God
> To Family
> To Authority

Law of Benevolence

> To Poor
> To Orphans/Widows
> To Servants

Law of Equity

> To Neighbor

ARRANGEMENT WORKSHEET

Refining the Case
& the Refutation II

Part One: Generate the Outline

1. Express your thesis in the form "Whether X should be punished for Y."

2. Generate your outline by completing the table below.

Prosecution	Defense
Evidence:	Argument I:
I.	I.
2.	2.
3.	3.
Law Broken	Argument 2:
I.	I.
2.	2.
3.	3.
Cause/Motive:	Argument 3:
I.	I.
2.	2.
3.	3.

103

Part 2: Generate the Refutation for the Prosecution

1. List the prosecution and defense arguments in the chart in part 3.

2. Refute the case for the defense. Record the answers in the chart in part 3.

Choose whether the case for the defense is arguing that:

☐ *There is not enough evidence to prove the defendant acted* (an sit)

☐ *Though the defendant acted, he did not break a law* (quid sit)

☐ *Though the defendant broke a law, he was excused or justified* (quale sit)

Part 3: Generate the Refutation for the Defense

Rebuild the case for the defense:

1. Summarize the case for the defense.

2. Explain why the prosecution fails to refute the case for the defense.

	Prosecution's Case	**Defense's Case**
Argument I:		
Argument 2:		
Argument 3:		
	Prosecution's Refutation	**Defense's Refutation**
Defense I:		
Why inadequate?		
Defense 2:		
Why inadequate?		
Prosecution's argument for inadequacy I		
Why is DI adequate?		
Prosecution's argument for inadequacy 2		
Why is D2 adequate?		

Add the appropriate refutation to your outline.

JUDICIAL ADDRESS SIX: ARRANGEMENT TEMPLATE

I. **Introduction**
   A. Kind of Exordium*
   B. Narratio
      1. Cause 1**
      2. Cause 2**
      3. Cause 3**
      4. Situation**
   C. Division
      1. Agreement*
      2. Disagreement
         a. Counter-Thesis*
         b. Thesis*
   D. Distribution
      1. Thesis*
      2. Enumeration*
      3. Exposition
         a. Argument I*
         b. Argument II*
         c. Argument III*

II. **Case**
   A. Argument I*
      1. Support 1*
      2. Support 2*
      3. Support 3*
      4. Kind of Terminating Sentence*
   B. Argument II*
      1. Support 1*
      2. Support 2*
      3. Support 3*
      4. Kind of Terminating Sentence*
   C. Argument III*
      1. Support 1*
      2. Support 2*
      3. Support 3*
      4. Kind of Terminating Sentence*

III. **Refutation**
   A. Counter-Thesis*
   B. Counter-Argument I*
      1. Summary of support for Counter-Argument I*
      2. Inadequacy of Counter-Argument I*
   C. Counter-Argument II*
      1. Summary of support for Counter-Argument II*
      2. Inadequacy of Counter-Argument II*
   D. Summary of Refutation*

IV. **Conclusion**
   A. Thesis*
   B. Summary of Case
      1. Argument I*
      2. Argument II*
      3. Argument III*
   C. Amplification
      1. What does the judge care about?*
      2. How will it be affected?*

ELOCUTION WORKSHEET A

Hyperbole

Key Terms:

◇ **Hyperbole:** A trope that emphasizes an idea by exaggerating it to an unreal or impossible proportion.

Examples from Great Literature

William Shakespeare's *Antony and Cleopatra*, Act V, Scene III

Let Rome in Tiber melt and the wide arch
Of the rang'd empire fall! Here is my space.

Ralph Waldo Emerson's "The Concord Hymn"

Here once the embattled farmers stood
And fired the **shot heard round the world**.

W.H. Auden's "As I Walked Out One Evening"

I'll love you dear, I'll love you
Till China and Africa meet,
And the river jumps over the mountain
And the salmon sing in the street.

Kenneth Grahame's "The Song of Toad"

But **never a name to go down in fame**,
Compared with that of Toad.
The clever men at Oxford
Know all that there is to be knowed.

Steps to Write Hyperbole

1. Select a specific characteristic to emphasize.

2. Identify the measurable quantity expressed in the characteristic.

3. Push that measurable quantity to an utterly unrealistic degree or proportion.

4. Rewrite the sentence by incorporating the unrealistic quantity.

Practice

1. Write hyperbole for a tool or toy you use or have used:

Characteristic:

_____

Measurable quantity:

_____

Unrealistic degree:

_____

Sentence:

_____

2. Write hyperbole for something you can find in your imagination:

Characteristic:

_____

Measurable quantity:

_____

Unrealistic degree:

_____

Sentence:

_____

3. Write hyperbole for something from a story:

Characteristic:

_____

Measurable quantity:

_____

Unrealistic degree:

_____

Sentence:

_____

4. Add hyperbole to your address.

ELOCUTION WORKSHEET B

Litotes

Key Terms:

◇ **Litotes:** A trope that negates the opposite characteristic of a term.

Examples from Great Literature

Bible, Acts 21:39

I am a Jew, from Tarsus of Cilicia, a citizen of **no mean city.**

Jonathan Swift's *A Tale of Tub*

I am not unaware how the productions of the Grub Street brotherhood have of late fallen under many prejudices.

Bible, Jeremiah 30:19

And out of them shall proceed thanksgiving and the voice of them that make merry: and I will multiply them, **and they shall not be few...**

Samuel Johnson's *Adventurer* No. 138

To write is indeed, **no unpleasing employment.**

Steps to Write Litotes

1. Select a sentence to emphasize.

2. Select a characteristic, quantity, or quality in the sentence to emphasize.

3. State the opposite of the characteristic, quantity, or quality. Do not say "no" or "not."

4. Add a negative to the opposite.

5. Rewrite the sentence using the new phrase.

Practice

1. Write litotes for a tool or toy you use or have used:

Characteristic:

_____

Opposite:

_____

Negated opposite:

_____

Sentence:

_____

2. Write litotes for something you can find in your imagination:

Characteristic:

_____

Opposite:

___

Negated opposite:

___

Sentence:

___

3. Write litotes for something from a story:

Characteristic:

___

Opposite:

___

Negated opposite:

___

Sentence:

___

4. Add litotes to your address.

Additional Elocution Practice

Level I Schemes: parallelism, antithesis, alliteration, assonance
Level I Tropes: simile, metaphor
Level II Schemes: compound sentences, complex sentences, anaphora,
epistrophe, sentence amplification
Level II Tropes: personification, apostrophe, synecdoche, hyperbole, litotes

On a separate sheet of paper write . . .

1. An example of parallelism

2. An example of antithesis

3. An example of alliteration

4. An example of assonance

5. An example of simile

6. An example of metaphor

7. An example of personification

8. An example of apostrophe

9. An example of a compound sentence

10. An example of a complex sentence

11. An example of anaphora

12. An example of epistrophe

13. An example of an amplified sentence

14. An example of synechdoche

Add at least two of the schemes and/or tropes you reviewed to your address.

Also add hyperbole and litotes.

JUDICIAL ADDRESS SEVEN

JUDICIAL ADDRESS SEVEN

Invention Review

The following worksheet is found in the Student Workbook on page 116, but is also ideal for in-class review and discussion.

Review the following

Character bias
Justice
An Sit
Quid Sit
Quale Sit

1. Demonstrate how to use each of the topics of Invention:

_____

_____

_____

_____

2. Describe how you use each:

_____

_____

_____

_____

3. Begin a judicial address using the tools learned.

JUDICIAL ADDRESS SEVEN

Arrangement Review

The following worksheet is found in the Student Workbook on page 117, but is also ideal for in-class review and discussion.

1. List the elements of a judicial address:

_____

_____

_____

_____

2. Generate an example of each element:

_____

_____

_____

_____

3. Explain how you construct each element of Arrangement:

_____

_____

_____

_____

4. Generate an outline for your judicial address.

COMPLETE JUDICIAL ADDRESS ARRANGEMENT TEMPLATE

Introduction
    A. Kind of Exordium*
    B. Narratio
          1. Cause 1**
          2. Cause 2**
          3. Cause 3**
          4. Situation**
    C. Division
          1. Agreement*
          2. Disagreement
               a. Counter-Thesis*
               b. Thesis*
    D. Distribution
          1. Thesis*
          2. Enumeration*
          3. Exposition
               a. Argument I*
               b. Argument II*
               c. Argument III*

I.   Case
    A. Argument I*
          1. Support 1*
          2. Support 2*
          3. Support 3*
          4. Kind of Terminating Sentence*
    B. Argument II*
          1. Support 1*
          2. Support 2*
          3. Support 3*
          4. Kind of Terminating Sentence*
    C. Argument III*
          1. Support 1*
          2. Support 2*
          3. Support 3*
          4. Kind of Terminating Sentence*

II.   Refutation
    A. Counter-Thesis*
    B. Counter-Argument I*
          1. Summary of support for Counter-Argument I*
          2. Inadequacy of Counter-Argument I*
    C. Counter-Argument II*
          1. Summary of support for Counter-Argument II*
          2. Inadequacy of Counter-Argument II*
    D. Summary of Refutation*

III.   Conclusion
    A. Thesis*
    B. Summary of Case
          1. Argument I*
          2. Argument II*
          3. Argument III*
    C. Amplification
          1. What does the judge care about?*
          2. How will it be affected?*

ELOCUTION WORKSHEET A
Erotema

Key Terms:

◊ **Erotema:** A trope in which a question is asked but no answer is expected.

Examples from Great Literature

Harper Lee's *To Kill a Mockingbird*

If there's just one kind of folks, **why can't they get along with each other?**

Patrick Henry's "Give Me Liberty or Give Me Death" speech

Why stand we here idle?
What is it that Gentlemen wish?

Mark Twain's *An Author's Soldiering*

Do you sense the whole magnitude of this conjunction, and perceive with what opulence of blessing for this nation it is freighted? What is it we are doing?

E.C. Stanton's *The Solitude of Self*

Such is individual life. **Who, I ask you, can take, dare take, on himself, the rights, the duties, the responsibilities, of another human soul?**

John C. Calhoun's *Nullification and the Force Bill*

Who ever heard of the United State of New York, of Massachusetts, or of Virginia? Who ever heard the term federal or union applied to the aggregation of individuals into one community?

William Shakespeare's *Hamlet*, Act IV, Scene V

O heavens! **Is't possible a young maid's wits**
Should be as mortal as an old man's life?

Steps to Write Erotema

1. Choose a declarative statement.

2. Rephrase the declarative statement as a question.

Practice

1. Choose a declarative statement:

_____

2. Rephrase the declarative statement as a question that elicits the desired conclusion:

_____

_____

_____

3. Add erotema to your address.

ELOCUTION WORKSHEET B

Hypophora

Key Terms:

◇ **Hypophora:** A trope in which a question is asked and immediately answered.

Examples from Great Literature

Christina Rossetti's "Who Hath Seen the Wind?"

Who hath seen the wind?
Neither you nor I.

William Shakespeare's "Sonnet 18"

Shall I compare thee to a summer's day?
Thou art more lovely and more temperate

Christina Rossetti's "What are Heavy? Sea-sand and Sorrow"

What are heavy? **Sea-sand and sorrow:**
What are brief? **Today and tomorrow:**
What are frail? **Spring blossoms and youth:**
What are deep? **The ocean and truth.**

Patrick Henry's "The Necessity of War"

Are we disposed to be of the number of those who, having eyes, see not and, having ears, hear not the things which so nearly concern their temporal salvation? **For my part, whatever anguish of spirit it may cost, I am willing to know the whole truth; to know the worst and to provide for it.**

Bible, Psalm 42:5

Why are you cast down, O my soul?
Hope thou in God.

Steps to Write Hypophora

1. Choose a declarative statement.

2. Rephrase the declarative statement as a question that elicits the desired conclusion and state the answer in simple terms.

Practice

1. Choose a declarative statement:

_____

2. Rephrase the declarative statement as a question that elicits the desired conclusion and state the answer in simple terms:

_____

_____

_____

3. Add hypophora to your address.

Additional Elocution Practice

Level I Schemes: parallelism, antithesis, alliteration, assonance
Level I Tropes: simile, metaphor
Level II Schemes: compound sentences, complex sentences, anaphora, epistrophe, sentence amplification
Level II Tropes: personification, apostrophe, synecdoche, hyperbole, litotes, erotema, hypophora

On a separate sheet of paper write . . .

1. An example of parallelism

2. An example of antithesis

3. An example of alliteration

4. An example of assonance

5. An example of simile

6. An example of metaphor

7. An example of personification

8. An example of apostrophe

9. An example of a compound sentence

10. An example of a complex sentence

11. An example of anaphora

12. An example of epistrophe

13. An example of an amplified sentence

14. An example of synechdoche

15. An example of hyperbole

16. An example of litotes

Add at least two of the schemes and/or tropes you reviewed to your address.
Also add erotema and hypohora.

APPENDICES

Appendix One: Tools of Invention

Definition	Definition	A common topic that states the limits within which a word has meaning.
	Procedure	Identify the category to which a thing belongs, compare it to other members of that set, identify its parts or aspects, and identify what differentiates it from other members of the set.
	Example	George Washington was the first president under the current U.S. Constitution.
Comparison	Definition	A common topic that asks how two terms are similar and different.
	Procedure	Select two terms and determine similarities and differences by asking what they both "have," "are," and "do."
	Example	Odysseus and the Sirens are both living creatures far from Ithaka, both have desires and companions, and both sing and want something, but are different in kind because Odysseus desires to go home while the Sirens desire the flesh of men, and they are different in degree because Odysseus is temporarily far from Ithaka while the Sirens are permanently far from Ithaka.
Circumstance	Definition	A common topic that describes the actions and events that occur at the same time as (but in different locations from) the situation of the issue.
	Procedure	Identify the time and place of the situation in the issue, then ask what is happening there, what is happening just outside of that location, and what is happening farther outside that location.
	Example	When Odysseus passes the Sirens, he is tied to the mast of his ship, his men have their ears stopped, his wife is being overrun by suitors in Ithaka, and his son is visiting the homes of Nestor and Menelaus.
Relation	Definition	A common topic that lists events or actions that take place before and after the situation of the issue and determines which are causes and which are effects.
	Procedure	Describe the situation of the issue, list several actions or events that preceded the situation, circle those that caused the situation, then list several actions or events that followed the situation, and circle those that were caused by the situation.
	Example	Before becoming president, George Washington was a general and fought in the Revolutionary War (his fame as a general caused him to become president). After his presidency, he stepped down after two terms and retired to his farm (he stepped down because of his presidency).
Testimony	Definition	A common topic that asks witnesses what they know about the situation or the event.
	Procedure	Name an eyewitness, character witness, or expert witness, identify what they would say about the situation, and consider their reliability. In Level II, reliability will be partly judged based on any bias they might have.
	Example	George Washington's father is an eyewitness to George's honesty after George confessed he damaged his father's cherry tree. He is somewhat reliable because he is biased in favor of his son's reputation.
Justice	Definition	A special topic that asks if the action of issue was right, fair, or appropriate.
	Procedure	Describe the situation of the issue and ask in what way the action was right, fair, or inappropriate.
	Example	Odysseus being tied to the mast and listening to the Sirens was just because there was no legal or moral prohibition against it and he was doing what the gods had said he could.
An Sit	Definition	A special topic used to collect evidence to determine whether an act occurred and whether the defendant committed the act.
	Procedure	Ask what evidence indicates that the action happened and what evidence indicates that the defendant committed the act, then ask if the evidence is reliable or credible.
	Example	The blood on Brutus' hands indicates he was at Caesar's murder, and the quantity of blood further indicates he was close to Caesar at the time.

Quid Sit	Definition	A special topic used to discover what happened and whether a law was violated.
	Procedure	Ask what rules were broken and kept, and ask what harms resulted or were prevented.
	Example	Scout disobeyed Atticus by crawling under the Radley fence and caused Nathan to fire his shotgun to scare off an intruder.
Quale Sit	Definition	A special topic used to discover why a defendant committed an act and whether the act is justifiable or excusable.
	Procedure	Ask what caused the defendant to commit the act, and ask if there are any reasons the action might be excused or justified.
	Example	Brutus killed Caesar because Caesar was too ambitious, and Brutus was trying to save Rome from a potential tyrant.

Appendix Two: Elements of Arrangement

Amplification	Definition	The extension or an enlargement of an idea or element. It can be used with a sentence, a paragraph, or an element of Arrangement, such as the conclusion. In LTW I, it was used with the conclusion. In LTW II, it is used with the conclusion and with sentences.
	Procedure	Identify additional information that will increase the impact of an idea and add it to the sentence or conclusion. In the conclusion, this information is who cares and why, or, in LTW II, who does the audience care about and how will they be affected by the audience's decision. For a sentence, students add an additional clause that expands the idea.
	Example	LTW I conclusion: The American colonists will be greatly affected by this decision, as it could lead a future tyrant taking power in the United States. LTW II conclusion: If you punish Jem for the death of Bob Ewell, Scout will grow up without a brother, alone and afraid. Sentence: Scout is a brave and curious young girl, a young girl who will not be embarrassed by any boy.
Argument	Definition	One of the three main points in the case section of a judicial address.
	Procedure	Identify the three strongest points from the PDI for either the prosecution or defense; each point is an argument.
	Example	The first reason Scout should be punished for crawling under the Radley fence is that the evidence is overwhelming that she did it.
Case	Definition	The argument of the judicial address, made up of the three arguments. In LTW I, this section was referred to as the proof section.
	Procedure	Identify the three strongest arguments from the PDI for either the prosecution or defense.
	Example	The first reason Scout should be punished for crawling under the Radley fence is that the evidence is overwhelming that she did it. The second reason Scout should be punished for crawling under the Radley fence is that she violated the local trespassing statute in doing so. The third reason Scout should be punished for crawling under the Radley fence is that she had cause and motive for doing so.
Division	Definition	A precise statement of the agreement and disagreement between the writer and an opponent.
	Procedure	Identify the thesis and the counter-thesis, what both sides agree on, and the precise point of disagreement.
	Example	While everyone agrees Scout crawled under the Radley fence, some believe she should be punished for it, while others believe she should not be.
Exordium	Definition	The opening of an essay, speech, or address, placed at the beginning of the introduction. Its purpose is to make the audience receptive to reading or listening.
	Procedure	Identify the audience's bias and explain why the bias should not prevent them from listening, using paradox, anecdote, or clarification.
	Example	"Friends, Romans, countrymen, lend me your ears; I come to bury Caesar, not to praise him." *Julius Caesar,* Act III, Scene 2
Narratio	Definition	Narrative; also called a "statement of facts" or "statement of circumstances." It tells a story, with settings, actors, and actions, to inform the reader of circumstances leading up to and causing the action that is the subject of the thesis.
	Procedure	Identify the setting and actors. Identify what caused the action in question. Identify what caused that, and so on as needed.
	Example	Cassius believed Caesar was ambitious, so he wanted to kill Caesar. His conspiracy needed a nobleman to give it credibility, so he invited Brutus, an honorable man, to join the cause. Brutus became persuaded of Caesar's ambition, so he agreed to participate. Together, they and the other conspirators went to the Senate on the Ides of March.

Proof	Definition	The particular reasons that make up the argument of essay in LTW I. The term is replaced by "case" in the judicial address when referring to the body and by "argument" when referring to the individual reasons in the body.
	Procedure	Identify the strongest reasons from the ANI and use them to prove the thesis.
	Example	The first reason Scout should not have crawled under the fence is that Jem was mocking her. The second reason Scout should not have crawled under the fence is that Atticus had forbidden her. The third reason Scout should not have crawled under the fence is that Nathan hadn't invited her.
Refutation	Definition	The response to an opposing argument.
	Procedure	Anticipate two arguments the opponent will make, state the two counter-proofs and explain why they are inadequate. In LTW II, the prosecution will proceed as above. The defense explains why the prosecution's refutation (his reasons the defense's case is inadequate) is not convincing. The defense simply rebuilds his own case.
	Example	Prosecution: Some say the blood on Brutus' hands does not prove he stabbed Caesar because it could have been splattered on him from a distance. This is an inadequate response because the quantity of blood indicates that he was very close, a sword handle's length away at most. Defense: Some have argued that the quantity of blood on Brutus' hands indicate he must have stabbed Caesar, but all it indicates is that he was close, close enough to have caught Caesar's body as it was falling to the floor, or even slipped in the blood himself.

Appendix Four: Tools of Elocution

Alliteration	Definition	A scheme repeating the same beginning consonants in three or more adjacent words.
	Procedure	Choose one word to emphasize in a supporting point. Note the consonant sound that the word begins with. Think of more words that start with that sound. Choose some and rewrite the sentence using three consecutive words that begin with the same sound.
	Example	The water washed wistfully over the sand.
Anaphora	Definition	A scheme in which the same word or phrase is repeated at the beginning of successive phrases, clauses, or sentences.
	Procedure	Select an idea, word, or phrase to emphasize. List several things about that idea, word, or phrase. Use your list to write three phrases, clauses, or sentences that all begin with the same word or words.
	Example	Odysseus was cunning; Odysseus was brave; Odysseus was crafty.
Antithesis	Definition	Two contrasting ideas written in a parallel structure.
	Procedure	Identify an idea to emphasize. Find its opposite, or a contrasting idea. Then write the two contrasting ideas in structures that are parallel to each other.
	Example	"That's one small step for man, one giant leap for mankind." Neil Armstrong, stepping onto the moon's surface.
Apostrophe	Definition	Addressing a personified inanimate object, a deceased person, yourself, or an idea.
	Procedure	Speak to someone or something that will not answer you.
	Example	"O mighty Caesar! Dost thou lie so low? Are all thy conquests, glories, triumphs, spoils, Shrunk to this little measure?" Shakespeare, *Julius Caesar*, 3.1
Assonance	Definition	A scheme in which one vowel sound is repeated in adjacent or closely connected words.
	Procedure	List many words that have the same, middle vowel sound. Use some of the words in a sentence together.
	Example	"Where the waves grow sweet, Doubt not, Reepicheep, To find all you seek, There is the utter East." *The Voyage of the Dawn Treader*
Epistrophe	Definition	A scheme in which the same word or phrase is repeated at the end of successive phrases, clauses, or sentences.
	Procedure	Find words to emphasize at the end of a sentence. Write more phrases using the same words at the end. Choose at least three to write in your essay.
	Example	"Government of the people, by the people, for the people..." Gettysburg Address
Hyperbole	Definition	A trope that makes a point by exaggerating an idea to an impossible or unreal proportion.
	Procedure	Find a quantity of something to emphasize. Rewrite the point as something or some amount that is exaggerated to an impossible number of items, places, etc.
	Example	"...the shot heard round the world" Ralph Waldo Emerson

Hypophora	Definition	A trope in which a question is asked and then answered afterwards.
	Procedure	Find a statement. Create some questions that your statement might be answering. Choose one question. Add the question to your essay, using the original statement as its answer.
	Example	"What made me take this trip to Africa? There is no quick explanation. Things got worse and worse and worse and pretty soon they were too complicated." *A Christmas Memory* by Truman Capote
Litotes	Definition	Emphasizing a point by negating its opposite
	Procedure	Find a trait to emphasize. Find the opposite of that trait. Write a new sentence with a description that says your idea is not the opposite of the original trait.
	Example	Julius Caesar was not a dishonorable man.
Metaphor	Definition	A trope that indirectly (i.e., not using "like" or "as") compares two things that are different in kind but that share a similar trait.
	Procedure	Find a word or idea to emphasize. Identify a trait you want to point out. Find something else that has the same trait but is a different kind of thing. State that one thing IS the other thing.
	Example	"I am the vine, ye are the branches." John 15:5
Parallelism	Definition	Sentence structure that lines up parts of speech the same way in a series of words, phrases, or clauses.
	Procedure	Identify a statement with a good structure. Rewrite two words, phrases, or clauses that go with it, shaping their structures to be the same as the original word, phrase, or clause—often used in the three main reasons of a discourse.
	Example	Aeneas' identity demands his action, his action magnifies his reputation, and his reputation opens his future.
Personification	Definition	A trope in which human characteristics are attributed to an inanimate object.
	Procedure	Identify an object. Rewrite the sentence so that the object acts in a way that only a human can act.
	Example	"Have you not made a universal shout, That Tiber trembled underneath her banks, To hear the replication of your sounds Made in her concave shores?" Shakespeare, *Julius Caesar*, 1.1
Erotema	Definition	A trope that asks a question in order to elicit a specific response. It is designed to subtly influence the response the writer wishes to obtain from his audience. In its simplest form, the answer will be either "yes" or "no."
	Procedure	Find a statement to emphasize. Rewrite it as a question that calls for a "yes" or "no" answer.
	Example	"If you prick us, do we not bleed? If you poison us, do we not die? And if you wrong us, shall we not revenge?" Shakespeare, *The Merchant of Venice*, 3.1
Simile	Definition	A trope that explicitly compares two things that are different in kind but similar in some trait.
	Procedure	Find a word or idea to emphasize. Identify a trait you want to point out. Find something that shares that trait but is a different kind of thing. State that one thing is like the other.
	Example	"Edmund saw the drop for a second in midair, shining like a diamond." *The Lion, the Witch, and the Wardrobe*

Synecdoche	Definition	A trope in which a part of a thing or group is used to represent, or name, the whole thing.
	Procedure	Choose an idea to emphasize. List the parts of that thing or person. Choose one part to represent the whole.
	Example	"Take thy face hence." Shakespeare, *Macbeth*, 5.3

Appendix Five: Sample Addresses

The following sample addresses are rudimentary examples of what each address might look like with each of the requisite elements if written by a middle school student. These are not meant to be the highest form of each address and are basic examples. Please assess accordingly. The addresses may not match the sample worksheets in the guide because students do have the right to change their content between the time they create their outline and the time they write their address.

Complete Persuasive Essay: Sample A

Whether Brutus should have killed Julius Caesar

"Et tu, Brute?" Caesar groaned when he saw Brutus lift his sword against him, releasing his last breath with his blood. In Shakespeare's *Julius Caesar,* several Romans conspire to kill Caesar because they think he is a tyrant destined to destroy the Roman Republic. Among them are Brutus and Cassius.

Everyone agrees that Brutus killed Caesar, though some believe he should have, and others that he should not have. Brutus should not have killed Caesar for three reasons: Brutus' presumption, Caesar's person, and Portia's favor.

The first reason Brutus should not have killed Caesar is Brutus' presumption. Brutus was not acting wisely. Instead, his supposed friend, Cassius, was deceiving him. Through Cassius' machinations, Brutus agreed to kill Caesar because he might become a tyrant, not because he already was one. Brutus claimed to participate in the conspiracy out of his love for Rome, but it was this very love that should have prevented him from assassinating Caesar.

The second reason Brutus should not have killed Caesar is Caesar's person. Julius Caesar was a friend to Brutus. Furthermore, Caesar was a husband whose wife loved him and begged him not to go to the Senate that day from fear for his fate. I resist mentioning that Caesar was also the acclaimed ruler of the Republic. For Brutus to kill his friend, depriving a wife of her husband and the republic of its leader, was a dishonorable and immoral act.

The third reason Brutus should not have killed Caesar is Portia's favor. Portia was Brutus' wife. The night before the assassination, she had asked Brutus to share with her his dealings with these strange men, the conspirators. Portia would not have approved Brutus' plan, but he never listened to her. Her disapproval was so great that, though she was pregnant, she fell on her sword in the aftermath. The pregnant Portia, bringing life into the world, fell prey to Brutus' decision to bring death into the world.

Some people say Brutus should have killed Caesar because killing tyrants is just. Others have done it in the past and been praised for it, including Brutus' ancestor and father-in-law, and even characters in the Bible, like Jael. This argument is inadequate, however, because there is no proof that Caesar was or would become a tyrant. Brutus was speculating, like a gambler risking everything on the roulette wheel and losing.

Others say Brutus should have killed Caesar because doing so would save the Republic. The assassination would prevent Caesar's tyranny and allow Rome to continue as a republic. This argument is inadequate, too, because the Republic was so fragile after a century of civil wars that the assassination of Caesar finally killed it rather than save it.

Neither of these arguments–that Caesar was a tyrant or that the Republic would be saved–justify Brutus' brutal and faithless execution of Julius Caesar.

Brutus should not have killed Caesar because of his own presumption, Caesar's person, and Portia's favor. American citizens hear a great caution in Caesar's assassination because, like all civilized people, they prefer order to chaos and understand that assassinations cause chaos.

Complete Persuasive Essay: Sample Essay B

Whether Scout should have crawled under the fence

"Scout, I'm tellin' you for the last time, shut your trap or go home–I declare to the Lord you're gettin' more like a girl every day!" Jem yells these words to his younger sister on the night they decide to disobey their dad and sneak into Boo Radley's yard.

Scout, her brother Jem, and their friend Dill wondered about their mysterious neighbor, Boo Radley, all summer. Because Boo never left his house, the three of them would have had to sneak into his yard if they hoped to discover whether the rumors of Boo Radley's insanity were true. So on the last night of summer, they crawled under the fence like rabbits to get a closer look. After meeting Boo, Scout saw the kind of man he was and they became friends.

Everyone agrees that Scout crawled under the fence. However, some say Scout should have crawled under the fence, and others say she should not have. Scout should have crawled under the fence for three reasons: She was brave, she was adventurous, and she was curious.

The first reason Scout should have crawled under the fence is she was brave. Even though she was only five at the beginning of the book, she fought older boys and wasn't afraid to speak her mind. She even challenged the hypocrisy of her teacher who condemned prejudice but showed it toward blacks. Scout wasn't afraid of other people and showed that she wanted to form her own opinions. She was a lion, not afraid of others who were larger than she was.

The second reason Scout should have crawled under the fence is she was adventurous. While all the other girls in her neighborhood were wearing dresses and drinking tea at home, Scout was out climbing trees with Dill and Jem. She even wore pants so that she could always be ready for an adventure. She was used to exploring, so it wasn't hard for her to try this adventure also.

The third reason Scout should have crawled under the fence is she was curious. Scout asked her dad many questions throughout the book and always wanted to find the answers. When the trial began, she did everything she could to learn the truth of the accusations. If she hadn't crawled under the fence with Jem and Dill that night, she would have found another way to discover the truth of Boo Radley, and maybe that would have been more dangerous. Crawling under the fence was the best way to find the answers.

Some say Scout should not have crawled under the fence because she was a vulnerable young girl. However, she also had Dill and Jem with her, who were both older boys. Others say Scout should not have crawled under the fence because it was dangerous. She could have gotten in trouble, because trespassing on a dark night can make you look like a thief. However, Boo Radley was friendly, so she wasn't really in danger. Scout had two older boys with her, and the Radleys knew them and were kind. So she wasn't vulnerable or in any real danger.

Scout should have crawled under the fence because she was brave, she was adventurous, and she was curious. Boo cared whether Scout, Jem, and Dill crawled under the fence; he would not have been able to show them kindness otherwise.

Judicial Address One: Sample Address A

Whether Brutus should Have killed Julius Caesar

"Et tu, Brute?" Julius Caesar groaned when he saw Brutus lift his sword against him, releasing his last breath with his blood. Cassius had conspired to kill Caesar, but he needed the help of a highly respected comrade, to whom he and a number of co-conspirators subtly had presented his plan. Through his efforts, Brutus was persuaded. The following morning, the whole faction went to Pompey's Theater, where the Senate was meeting. There Brutus, Cassius, and the conspirators confronted Caesar and Brutus had to decide whether to fulfill the plan and execute the ruler of Rome.

Everyone agrees that Brutus killed Caesar, though some believe he should have, and others that he should not have. Brutus should not have killed Caesar for three reasons: his presumption, Caesar's person, and Portia's favor.

The first reason Brutus should not have killed Caesar is Brutus' presumption. Brutus was not acting wisely. Instead, his supposed friend, Cassius, was deceiving him. Through Cassius' machinations, Brutus agreed to kill Caesar because he might become a tyrant, not because he already was one. Brutus claimed to participate in the conspiracy out of his love for Rome, but it was this very love that should have prevented him from assassinating Caesar.

The second reason Brutus should not have killed Caesar is Caesar's person. Julius Caesar was a friend to Brutus. Furthermore, Caesar was a husband whose wife loved him and begged him not to go to the Senate that day from fear for his fate. For Brutus to kill his friend, depriving a wife of her husband and the republic of a leader, was a dishonorable and immoral act.

The third reason Brutus should not have killed Caesar is Portia's favor. Portia was Brutus' wife. The night before the assassination, she had asked Brutus to share with her his dealings with these strange men, the conspirators. Portia would not have approved Brutus' plan, but he never listened to her. Oh, sword! You rushed too quickly to the Capitol. Her disapproval was so great that, though she was pregnant, she fell on her sword in the aftermath. The pregnant Portia, bringing life into the world, fell prey to Brutus' decision to bring death into the world.

Some people say Brutus should have killed Caesar because killing tyrants is just. Others have done it in the past and been praised for it, including Brutus's ancestor and father-in-law, and even characters in the Bible, like Jael. This argument is inadequate, however, because there is no proof that Caesar was or would become a tyrant. Brutus was speculating, like a gambler risking everything on the roulette wheel and losing.

Others say Brutus should have killed Caesar because doing so would save the Republic. The assassination would prevent Caesar's tyranny and allow Rome to continue as a republic. The crown had not yet ascended the throne of his head. This argument is inadequate, too, because the Republic was so fragile after a century of civil wars that the assassination of Caesar finally killed it, rather than saving it.

Neither of these arguments–that Caesar was a tyrant or that the Republic would be saved–justify Brutus' brutal and faithless execution of Julius Caesar.

Brutus should not have killed Caesar because of his own presumption, Caesar's person, and Portia's favor. American citizens hear a great caution in Caesar's assassination because, like all civilized people, they prefer order to chaos and understand that assassinations cause chaos.

Judicial Address One: Sample Address B

Whether Scout should have crawled under the fence

"Scout, I'm tellin' you for the last time, shut your trap or go home–I declare to the Lord you're gettin' more like a girl every day!" Jem yells these words to his younger sister on the night they decide to disobey their dad and sneak into Boo Radley's yard. Scout really wanted Jem and Dill's respect, so she wanted to prove Jem wrong.

Scout, her brother Jem, and their friend Dill had wondered about their mysterious neighbor, Boo Radley, all summer. Because Boo never left his house, the three of them had to sneak into his yard if they hoped to discover whether the rumors of Boo Radley's insanity were true. So on the last night of summer, Jem made fun of Scout, and they crawled under the fence like rabbits to get a closer look. After meeting Boo, Scout saw his sanity and they became friends.

Everyone agrees that trespassing is dangerous. So, some say Scout should have crawled under the fence, while others say she shouldn't have. Scout should have crawled under the fence for three reasons: She was brave, she was adventurous, and she was curious.

The first reason Scout should have crawled under the fence is that she was brave. Even though she was only five at the beginning of the book, she fought older boys and wasn't afraid to speak her mind. She even challenged the hypocrisy of her teacher who condemned prejudice but showed it toward blacks. Scout wasn't afraid of other people, and showed that she wanted to form her own opinions. She was a lion, not afraid of others who were larger than she was.

The second reason Scout should have crawled under the fence is that she was adventurous. While all the other girls in her neighborhood were wearing dresses and drinking tea at home, Scout was out climbing trees with Dill and Jem. She even wore pants so that she could always be ready for an adventure. She was used to exploring, so it wasn't be hard for her to try this adventure also. **Come on, feet, take Scout somewhere new.**

The third reason Scout should have crawled under the fence is that she was curious. Scout asked her dad many questions throughout the book and always wanted to find the answers. When the trial began, she did everything she could to learn the truth of the accusations. If she had not crawled under the fence with Jem and Dill that night, she would have found another way to discover the truth of Boo Radley, and maybe that would have been more dangerous. **The house with its bright lights and empty porch was inviting them in.** Crawling under the fence was the best way to find the answers.

Some say Scout should not have crawled under the fence because she was a vulnerable young girl. However, she also had Dill and Jem with her, who were both older boys. Others say Scout should not have crawled under the fence because it was dangerous. She could have gotten in trouble, because trespassing on a dark night can make you look like a thief. However, Boo Radley was friendly, so she wasn't really in danger. Scout had two older boys with her, and the Radleys knew them and were kind. So she wasn't vulnerable or in any real danger.

Scout should have crawled under the fence because she was brave, she was adventurous, and she was curious. Boo cares whether Scout, Jem, and Dill crawl under the fence. He would not have been able to show them kindness otherwise.

Judicial Address Two: Sample Address A

Exordium with transition to narratio
Terminating sentences and citations

Whether Brutus should be punished for killing Julius Caesar

It is true that Brutus appears to be an honorable and wise man, but, hard as it is to accept, he was a cruel assassin. Prior to the Ides of March, Cassius had conspired to kill Caesar, but he needed the help of a highly respected comrade. They knew they needed Brutus, to whom he and a number of co-conspirators subtly presented his plan. Through his efforts, Brutus was persuaded. The following morning, the whole faction went to Pompey's Theater, where the Senate was meeting. There Brutus, Cassius, and the conspirators confronted Caesar, and Brutus had to decide whether to fulfill the plan and execute the ruler of Rome. He did.

Everyone agrees that Brutus killed Caesar, though some believe he should have, while others that he should not have. Brutus should not have killed Caesar for three reasons: Brutus' presumption, Caesar's person, and Portia's favor.

The first reason Brutus should not have killed Caesar is that Brutus was presumptuous. Brutus was not acting wisely. Instead, his supposed friend, Cassius, was deceiving him. Through Cassius' machinations, Brutus agreed to kill Caesar because he might become a tyrant, not because he already was one (*Julius Caesar*, III.I.121). Brutus claimed to participate in the conspiracy out of his love for Rome, but it was this very love that should have prevented him from assassinating Caesar. It is clear that Brutus was presumptuous in his decision.

The second reason Brutus should not have killed Caesar is Caesar's person. Julius Caesar was a friend to Brutus. Furthermore, Caesar was a husband whose wife loved him and begged him not to go to the Senate that day from fear for his fate. For Brutus to kill his friend, depriving a wife of her husband and the republic of a leader, was a dishonorable and immoral act. Caesar did not deserve such treatment from a friend.

The third reason Brutus should not have killed Caesar is Portia's favor. Portia was Brutus' wife. The night before the assassination, she had asked Brutus to share with her his dealings with these strange men, the conspirators. Portia would not have approved Brutus' plan, but he never listened to her. Oh, sword! You rushed too quickly to the Capitol. Her disapproval was so great that, though she was pregnant, she fell on her sword in the aftermath. The pregnant Portia, bringing life into the world, fell prey to Brutus' decision to bring death into the world (*Julius Caesar*, II.I.255-256). Portia deserved better from her husband.

Some people say Brutus should have killed Caesar because killing tyrants is just. Others have done it in the past and been praised for it, including Brutus' ancestor and father-in-law, and even characters in the Bible, like Jael. This argument is inadequate, however, because there is no proof that Caesar was or would become a tyrant. Brutus was speculating, like a gambler risking everything on the roulette wheel and losing.

Others say Brutus should have killed Caesar because doing so would save the Republic. The assassination prevented Caesar's tyranny and allowed Rome to continue as a republic. The crown had not yet ascended the throne of his head. This argument is inadequate, too, because the Republic was so fragile after a century of civil wars that the assassination of Caesar finally killed it, rather than saving it.

Neither of these arguments—that Caesar was a tyrant or that the Republic could have been saved—justify Brutus' brutal and faithless execution of Julius Caesar.

Brutus should not have killed Caesar because of his own presumption, Caesar's person, and Portia's favor. American citizens hear a great caution in Caesar's assassination because, like all civilized people, they prefer order to chaos and understand that assassinations cause chaos.

Judicial Address Two: Sample Address B

Audience: Nathan Radley

Whether Scout should be punished for crawling under the Radley fence

Boo is an innocent and good person, but this is exactly the reason why Scout should not be punished. That night, Atticus had left Scout in Jem's care. Jem and Dill were busy bragging about their bravery to each other and daring each other to touch the Radley house. When Jem and Dill acted on each other's dares, Scout was dragged along to the Radley house.

Everyone agrees that trespassing is illegal. Some say Scout should be punished for crawling under the Radley fence, and others say she should not. Scout should not be punished for crawling under the Radley fence for three reasons: Jem and Dill made her go, Atticus told her to stay with Jem, and Boo was befriending her.

The first reason Scout should not be punished for crawling under the Radley fence is that Jem and Dill made her go. Jem was Scout's older brother and was watching her. He, however, was busy daring Dill and wanted to go to the Radley house to prove his bravery. Scout tried to talk them out of it, but Jem and Dill simply made fun of her for acting like a girl (*To Kill a Mockingbird*, pg. 60). This helps us to see that Scout went against her will.

The second reason Scout should not be punished for crawling under the Radley fence is Atticus told her to stay with Jem. As above, Scout was obligated to remain with Jem. While it may appear that Scout was disobeying Atticus, who told her to leave the Radleys alone, Scout was actually obeying Atticus, who told her to stay with Jem. Scout had to choose between two conflicting commands. She chose the most recent one and obeyed it. Either Scout disobeyed Atticus by going to the Radleys or disobeyed Atticus by leaving Jem; she "had no option but to join them" (*To Kill a Mockingbird*, pg. 60).

The third reason Scout should not be punished for crawling under the Radley fence is that Boo was befriending her. Boo had been watching Scout, Jem, and Dill as they played and went on their little escapades (*To Kill a Mockingbird,* pg. 28). He had also been leaving little trinkets and toys in the knothole of a neighborhood tree, all gifts for Jem and Scout. Boo left these trinkets until you, Nathan, sealed up the hole, preventing any future gift-giving. A just person would not punish a little girl who was visiting a friend.

Some say Scout should be punished for crawling under the Radley fence because she was not invited. However, a person can visit a friend without an invitation and that would not be considered trespassing. Others say Scout should be punished for crawling under the Radley fence because she was disobeying Atticus. Scout may have disobeyed Atticus, but by not going with Jem and Dill she would also have been disobeying Atticus. She had no choice. Scout was visiting a friend and was obeying Atticus even while disobeying him. She does not deserve to be punished.

Scout should not be punished for crawling under the Radley fence because Jem and Dill made her go, Atticus told her to stay with Jem, and Boo was befriending her. Boo is an innocent and good person, who was friendly and kind to Scout. He would not want to see her punished for that night.

Judicial Address Three: Sample Address A

Refining the amplification
Compound and complex sentences

Whether Brutus should be punished for murdering Caesar

It is true that Brutus appears to be an honorable and wise man, but, hard as it is to accept, he was a cruel assassin. Prior to the Ides of March, Cassius had conspired to kill Caesar, but he needed the help of a highly respected comrade. They knew they needed Brutus, to whom Cassius and a number of co-conspirators subtly presented his plan. Through his efforts, Brutus was persuaded. The following morning, the whole faction went to Pompey's Theater, where the Senate was meeting. There Brutus, Cassius, and the conspirators confronted Caesar, and Brutus had to decide whether to fulfill the plan and execute the ruler of Rome. He did.

Everyone agrees that Brutus killed Caesar. While some believe Brutus should not be punished for murdering Caesar, others believe he should. Brutus should be punished for three reasons: Brutus' presumption, Caesar's person, and Portia's favor.

The first reason Brutus should be punished for murdering Caesar is that the evidence proves he did it. Brutus was a member of the conspiracy to kill Caesar, joining Cassius, Cinna, Casca, and others. Using his own sword, he stabbed Caesar. Since Brutus showed no remorse, he washed his hands in the blood of Caesar (*Julius Caesar*, III.I.118). All of this was seen by the Senators present and was openly confessed by Brutus himself. Clearly, the evidence shows he is guilty of murdering Caesar.

The second reason Brutus should be punished for murdering Caesar is that he violated the law. Natural law teaches to honor those in authority, and Roman laws forbade murder. Brutus murdered Caesar, a man with the highest authority in Rome. His actions violated both natural law and the laws of Rome. To break the law is to be guilty.

The third reason Brutus should be punished for murdering Caesar is that it caused many and great harms. Caesar lost his life, and he could no longer lead his country, love his wife, or father children.

Leaderless, Rome was cast into what became a three-way civil war between Brutus, Octavius, and Mark Antony. And for the coup de grace, Brutus himself became a tyrant. Such harms demand justice.

Some people say Brutus is not guilty of murdering Caesar because he kept a higher law: the preservation of the Roman Republic. Brutus' duty to the Republic, however, was as false as his honor. His love of glory and his desire for power led to the collapse of the Republic into civil war.

Others say Brutus is not guilty of murdering Caesar because it prevented greater harms. But it is hard to imagine worse harm than the ensuing civil war, the slaughter of many armies, and the end of the Republic for which Brutus claimed he was fighting. Neither of these arguments—that Brutus kept a higher law or that he prevented greater harms—justify Brutus's actions.

Brutus is guilty of murdering Caesar because the evidence is strong, he violated the law, and he caused many and great harms. Cicero would be indignant if the republic were to collapse into civil war should Brutus get away with the assassination.

Judicial Address Three: Sample Address B

Audience: Nathan Radley

Whether Scout should be punished for crawling under the Radley fence

Boo is an innocent and good person, but this is exactly the reason why Scout should not be punished. That night, Atticus had left Scout in Jem's care. Jem and Dill were busy bragging about their bravery to each other and daring each other to touch the Radley house. When Jem and Dill acted on each other's dares, Scout was dragged along to the Radley house.

Everyone agrees that trespassing is illegal. Some say Scout should be punished for crawling under the Radley fence, and others say she should not. Scout should not be punished for crawling under the Radley fence for three reasons: Jem and Dill made her go, Atticus told her to stay with Jem, and Boo was befriending her.

The first reason Scout should not be punished for crawling under the Radley fence is that Jem and Dill made her go. Jem was Scout's older brother and was watching her. He, however, was busy daring Dill and wanted to go to the Radley house to prove his bravery. Scout tried to talk them out of it, but Jem and Dill simply made fun of her for acting like a girl (*To Kill a Mockingbird*, pg. 60). This helps us to see that Scout went against her will.

The second reason Scout should not be punished for crawling under the Radley fence is that Atticus told her to stay with Jem. As above, Scout was obligated to remain with Jem. While it may appear that Scout was disobeying Atticus, who told her to leave the Radleys alone, Scout was actually obeying Atticus, who told her to stay with Jem. Scout had to choose between two conflicting commands. She chose the most recent one and obeyed it. While Scout disobeyed Atticus by going to the Radleys, she obeyed him by staying with Jem. She "had no option but to join them" (*To Kill a Mockingbird*, pg. 60).

The third reason Scout should not be punished for crawling under the Radley fence is Boo was befriending her. Boo had been watching Scout, Jem, and Dill as they played and went on their little escapades (*To Kill a Mockingbird*, pg. 28). He had also been leaving little trinkets and toys in the knothole of a neighborhood tree, all gifts for Jem and Scout. Boo left these trinkets until you, Nathan, sealed up the hole, preventing any future gift-giving. A just person would not punish a little girl who was visiting a friend.

Some say Scout should be punished for crawling under the Radley fence because she was not invited. However, a person can visit a friend without an invitation and that would not be considered trespassing. Others say Scout should be punished for crawling under the Radley fence because she was disobeying Atticus. Scout may have disobeyed Atticus, but by not going with Jem and Dill she would also have been disobeying Atticus. She had no choice. Scout was visiting a friend and was obeying Atticus even while disobeying him. She does not deserve to be punished.

Scout should not be punished for crawling under the Radley fence because Jem and Dill made her go, Atticus told her to stay with Jem, and Boo was befriending her. Boo is an innocent and good person, who was friendly and kind to Scout. By acquitting Scout, you ensure that Boo will have a friend and even that other neighbors may begin accepting him as part of the community.

Judicial Address Four: Sample Address A

An Sit
Anaphora and epistrophe

Whether Brutus killed Caesar

It is true that Brutus appears to be an honorable and wise man, but, hard as it is to accept, he was a cruel assassin. Prior to the Ides of March, Cassius had conspired to kill Caesar, but he needed the help of a highly respected comrade. They knew they needed Brutus, to whom he and a number of co-conspirators subtly presented his plan. Through his efforts, Brutus was persuaded. The following morning, the whole faction went to Pompey's Theater, where the Senate was meeting. There Brutus, Cassius, and the conspirators confronted Caesar, and Brutus had to decide whether to fulfill the plan and execute the ruler of Rome. He did.

Everyone agrees that Caesar was killed. Some contend Brutus did it, but others do not. Brutus did kill Caesar, as I will demonstrate through overwhelming evidence divided into three arguments: Brutus'sword, Caesar's body, and the witness of the Senators.

The first evidence that Brutus murdered Caesar is Brutus' sword. Brutus used his sword to stab Caesar. After the murder, it was covered in blood while still in Brutus' hand (*Julius Caesar*, III.I.121). This bloody sword belonged to Brutus and he used it to kill Caesar. The sword is clear evidence of Brutus' involvement.

The second evidence that Brutus murdered Caesar is Caesar's body. As Antony showed, Caesar's body was mangled by stab wounds and one of them was inflicted by Brutus. Bleeding from those wounds, Caesar died. The blood of Caesar was found on Brutus' hands. He was caught red-handed. Caesar's body, especially its blood on Brutus' hands, is clear evidence of Brutus' involvement.

The third evidence that Brutus murdered Caesar is the witness of the Senators. In the Capitol, Caesar and the conspirators were surrounded by senators who watched Brutus' foul act in horror. They heard Caesar cry, "Et tu, Brute?" They stared aghast as Brutus withdrew the sword from Caesar's body. They watched Brutus wash his hands in Caesar's blood (*Julius Caesar*, III.I.118). The senators' witness demonstrates Brutus' guilt.

The defense want to convince us that Brutus did not murder Caesar because the senators were biased against Brutus. And yet, all of the conspirators were Senators, and those who were not did nothing to stop them. Where do we see evidence of jealousy in the Senators? If anything, the Senators were inclined to favor Brutus.

The defense also want us to believe that Brutus was a victim of the chaos. Because he was standing nearby, he was covered in blood. But when Brutus presented his speech, he didn't talk like a bystander. He not only admitted he participated in the act, he not only tried to justify it, he not only slandered Caesar, he took the lead as representative for the conspirators.

Brutus murdered Caesar, as the evidence conclusively demonstrates: his sword boldly proclaimed that Brutus killed Caesar, the victim's body morbidly cried that Brutus killed Caesar, and the witness of the Senators meekly confessed that Brutus killed Caesar. The great advocate, Cicero, would be indignant if the republic were unable to convict so obvious a criminal.

Judicial Address Four: Sample Address B

Audience: Nathan Radley

Whether Scout crawled under the Radley fence

Note: this address is here to provide an example of a defense case. It is unlikely that one would take the defense position in an an sit address for Scout on this issue, since Scout, as narrator, admits to having crawled under the fence. This sample address is written out of necessity.

Boo is an innocent and good person, but that does not matter in this case. That night, Atticus had left Scout in Jem's care. Jem and Dill were busy bragging about their bravery to each other and daring each other to touch the Radley house. Scout was alone.

Everyone agrees that someone crawled under the Radley fence. Some say Scout crawled under the Radley fence, and others say she did not. It cannot be proved that Scout crawled under the Radley fence for three reasons: The pants were Jem's, the patch was on Jem's pants, and the gunshot was for a black man.

The first reason it cannot be proved that Scout crawled under the Radley fence is that the pants were Jem's (*To Kill a Mockingbird*, pg. 60). The prosecution believes that Jem's pants prove Scout's guilt. Jem's pants do not prove Scout was there, Jem's pants do not prove Dill was there, Jem's pants hardly prove he was there. Even if Jem were there, it would not necessitate that Scout was there with him. As a result, further evidence will be required to prove that Scout crawled under the Radley fence.

The second reason it cannot be proved that Scout crawled under the Radley fence is the patch was on Jem's pants. That there were pants at the scene, the prosecution has rightly noted. That there was a hole in the pants, the prosecution has rightly noted. That the hole was patched, the prosecution has rightly noted. As above, however, the patched pants belonged to Jem, and Jem's pants on the scene, patched or not, do not prove Scout was there. Even if you, Nathan, or your brother, Boo, put the patch there, it does not prove Scout was there. It is better to know that Scout was there than to find an innocent person guilty.

The third reason it cannot be proved that Scout crawled under the Radley fence is that the gunshot was for a black man. During the night in question, you fired your shotgun, Nathan. You reported to the neighborhood that you shot into the air to scare a black man from your collard patch (*To Kill a Mockingbird*, pg. 62). By your own admission, it was not Scout Finch who had crawled under your fence and was rooting around in your yard; it was a black man. It is rather difficult to believe that you confused an young, white girl for an adult black man. This is why it cannot be proved Scout crawled under the fence.

Some say the defense's argument that the pants belonged to Jem does not prove Scout was there is inadequate because Scout is always with Jem. While it is true that Scout is often with Jem, it is not true that she is always with Jem. When she is at school and when she is with Calpurnia are two obvious instances when she is not with Jem. Some say the defense's argument that you, Nathan, were scaring off a black man is inadequate because it was too dark to distinguish who was there. While it is true it was dark, making it difficult to identify features, that is precisely why it does not prove Scout was there. Thus, the evidence is insufficient to prove Scout crawled under the Radley fence.

It cannot be proved that Scout crawled under the Radley fence because the pants were Jem's, the patch was on Jem's pants, the gunshot was for a black man. Boo is an innocent and good person who was friendly and kind to Scout. By acquitting Scout, you ensure that Boo will have a friend and even that other neighbors may begin accepting him as part of the community.

Judicial Address Five: Sample Address A

Refining the case
Synecdoche and sentence amplification

Whether Brutus should be punished for murdering Caesar

It is true that Brutus appears to be an honorable and wise man, but, hard as it is to accept, he was a cruel assassin. Prior to the Ides of March, Cassius had conspired to kill Caesar, but he needed the help of a highly respected comrade. They knew they needed Brutus, to whom he and a number of co-conspirators subtly presented his plan. Through his efforts, Brutus was persuaded. The following morning, the whole faction went to Pompey's Theater, where the Senate was meeting. There Brutus, Cassius, and the conspirators confronted Caesar, and Brutus had to decide whether to fulfill the plan and execute the ruler of Rome. He did.

Everyone agrees that Brutus killed Caesar. While some believe Brutus should not be punished for murdering Caesar, others believe he should. Brutus should be punished for three reasons: the evidence of Brutus' sword, the evidence of Caesar's body, and the demands of the law.

The first reason Brutus should be punished for murdering Caesar is the evidence of Brutus' sword. Brutus used his sword to stab Caesar. After the murder, it was covered in blood while Brutus was still holding it (*Julius Caesar*, III.I.121). This bloody sword belonged to Brutus and he used it to kill Caesar. The sword is clear evidence of Brutus' involvement.

The second reason Brutus should be punished for murdering Caesar is the evidence of Caesar's body. As Antony showed, Caesar's body was mangled by stab wounds and one of them was inflicted by Brutus. Bleeding from those wounds, Caesar died. The blood of Caesar was found on Brutus' hands. He was caught red-handed. Caesar's body, especially its blood on Brutus' hands, is clear evidence of Brutus' guilt.

The third reason Brutus should be punished for murdering Caesar is that the law demands it. He broke the law that underlies every society: You must not murder, and you must especially not murder your rulers. Brutus had no excuse for his action, because he did it freely, without accident or compulsion. And he had no justification for his action because there is no higher law to which a murderer can appeal. Ten thousand tongues could not explain so great a crime.

Some people say Brutus is not guilty of murdering Caesar because he kept a higher law: the preservation of the Roman Republic. Brutus' duty to the Republic, however, was as false as his honor. His love of glory led him into folly and his desire for power led to the collapse of the Republic.

Others say Brutus is not guilty of murdering Caesar because the murder prevented greater harms. It is hard to imagine worse harm than the ensuing civil war, the slaughter of many armies, and the end of the Republic for which Brutus claimed he was fighting. Neither of these arguments—that Brutus kept a higher law or that he prevented greater harms—justify Brutus' actions.

Brutus should be punished for murdering Caesar because of the evidence of Brutus' sword, the evidence of Caesar's body, and the demands of the law. Cicero would be indignant if the republic were to collapse into civil war should Brutus get away with the assassination.

Judicial Address Five: Sample Address B

Audience: Nathan Radley

Whether Scout should be punished for trespassing

Boo is an innocent and good person, but this is exactly the reason why Scout should not be punished. That night, Atticus had left Scout in Jem's care. Jem and Dill were busy bragging about their bravery to each other and daring each other to touch the Radley house. When Jem and Dill acted on each other's dares, Scout was dragged along to the Radley house.

Everyone agrees that trespassing is illegal. Some say Scout should be punished for crawling under the Radley fence, and others say she should not. Scout should not be punished for crawling under the Radley fence for three reasons: Jem compelled her, she obeyed Atticus, and she honored a friend.

The first reason Scout should not be punished for crawling under the Radley fence is Jem compelled her. Jem was Scout's older brother and was watching her. He, however, was busy daring Dill and wanted to go to the Radley house to prove his bravery. Scout tried to talk them out of it, but Jem and Dill simply made fun of her for acting like a girl (*To Kill a Mockingbird*, pg. 60). This helps us to see that Scout went against her will.

The second reason Scout should not be punished for crawling under the Radley fence is that Atticus told her to stay with Jem. As above, Scout was obligated to remain with Jem. While it may appear that Scout was disobeying Atticus, who told her to leave the Radleys alone, Scout was actually obeying Atticus, who told her to stay with Jem. Scout had to choose between two conflicting commands. She chose the most recent one and obeyed it. I now realize that she "had no option but to join them" (*To Kill a Mockingbird*, pg. 60).

The third reason Scout should not be punished for crawling under the Radley fence is that she honored a friend. Boo had been watching Scout, Jem, and Dill as they played and went on their little escapades (*To Kill a Mockingbird*, pg. 28). He had also been leaving little trinkets and toys in the knothole of a neighborhood tree, all gifts for Jem and Scout. Boo left these trinkets until you, Nathan, sealed up the hole, preventing any future gift-giving. A just person would not punish the brave soul who was visiting her friend.

Some say the defense's argument that Scout obeyed Atticus is inadequate because Atticus told her to stay away from the Radleys, not to crawl under their fence. While it is true that Atticus gave her those instructions, they conflicted with his other instruction to stay with Jem. She obeyed the most recent command, after trying to dissuade Jem from going himself. Some say the defense's argument that Jem compelled Scout is inadequate because one is not compelled by name-calling. While it may be true that some people are not compelled by name-calling, Scout knew the name-calling carried with it other, more deleterious consequences. Thus, the prosecution's attack on the defense case is insufficient.

Scout should not be punished for crawling under the Radley fence because Jem compelled her, she obeyed Atticus, and she honored Boo. Boo is an innocent and good person, who was friendly and kind to Scout. By acquitting Scout, you ensure that Boo will have a friend and even that other neighbors may begin accepting him as part of the community.

Judicial Address Six: Sample Essay A

Refined case and refutation
Hyperbole and litotes

Whether Brutus should be punished for the murder of Julius Caesar

It is true that Brutus appears to be an honorable and wise man, but, hard as it is to accept, he was a cruel assassin. Prior to the Ides of March, Cassius had conspired to kill Caesar, but he needed the help of a highly respected comrade. They knew they needed Brutus, to whom he and a number of co-conspirators subtly presented his plan. Through his efforts, Brutus was persuaded. The following morning, the whole faction went to Pompey's Theater, where the Senate was meeting. There Brutus, Cassius, and the conspirators confronted Caesar, and Brutus had to decide whether to fulfill the plan and execute the ruler of Rome. He did.

Everyone agrees that Brutus killed Caesar. While some believe Brutus should not be punished for murdering Caesar, others believe he should. Brutus should be punished for three reasons: the evidence of Brutus' own words, the demands of the law, and the absence of a justification.

The first reason Brutus should be punished for murdering Caesar is the evidence of Brutus' own words. After the murder, Brutus mounted the rostrum and proclaimed to the Roman people that he and the other conspirators had killed Caesar. He was shameless in his confession, so much so that he brazenly allowed Antony to speak after him, thinking people would overlook his act because of his character. He was wrong. His confession should lead to his punishment.

The second reason Brutus should be punished for murdering Caesar is the demands of the law. He broke the law that underlies every society: You must not murder, and you must especially not murder your rulers. The law of nature prohibits murder, and Roman law going back to the *mos maiorum* had pronounced not the weakest penalties for such an evil deed.

The third reason Brutus should be punished for murdering Caesar is the absence of a justification. Brutus had no excuse for his action, because he did it freely, without accident or compulsion. He had motive: to be remembered as a hero like his ancestor. But he had no justification for his action because there is no higher law to which a murderer can appeal. Ten million tongues could not explain this horrific crime, the worst in all of world history.

Some people say Brutus should not be punished for murdering Caesar because he did keep a higher law: the preservation of the Roman Republic. Brutus' duty to the Republic, however, was as false as his honor. His love of glory led him into folly and his desire for power led to the collapse of the Republic. The idea that the Republic could be preserved by murdering its ruler is not an appeal to a higher law but the vain ravings of an unbalanced man.

Others say Brutus should not be punished for murdering Caesar because the murder prevented greater harms. It is hard to imagine a worse harm than the ensuing civil war, the slaughter of Roman armies, citizens, and even illustrious senators like Cicero, and the end of the Republic for which Brutus claimed he was fighting.

Neither of these arguments—that Brutus kept a higher law or that he prevented greater harms—justify Brutus' actions.

Brutus should be punished for murdering Caesar because of the evidence of Brutus' sword, the demands of the law, and the absence of justification. Cicero would be indignant if the republic were to collapse into civil war should Brutus get away with the assassination.

Judicial Address Six: Sample Address B

Audience: Nathan Radley

Whether Scout should be punished for trespassing

Boo is an innocent and good person, but this is exactly the reason why Scout should not be punished. That night, Atticus had left Scout in Jem's care. Jem and Dill were busy bragging about their bravery to each other and daring each other to touch the Radley house. When Jem and Dill acted on each other's dares, Scout was dragged along to the Radley house.

Everyone agrees that trespassing is illegal. Some say Scout should be punished for crawling under the Radley fence, and others say she should not. Scout should not be punished for crawling under the Radley fence for three reasons: Jem compelled her, she obeyed Atticus, and she honored a friend.

The first reason Scout should not be punished for crawling under the Radley fence is that Jem compelled her. Jem was Scout's older brother and was watching her. He, however, was busy daring Dill and wanted to go to the Radley house to prove he was braver than a lion. Scout tried to talk them out of it, but Jem and Dill simply made fun of her for acting like a girl (*To Kill a Mockingbird*, pg. 60). This helps us to see that Scout went against her will.

The second reason Scout should not be punished for crawling under the Radley fence is that Atticus told her to stay with Jem. As above, Scout was obligated to remain with Jem. While it may appear that Scout was disobeying Atticus, who told her to leave the Radleys alone, Scout was actually obeying Atticus, who told her to stay with Jem. Scout had to choose between two conflicting commands. She chose the most recent one and obeyed it. I now realize that she "had no option but to join them" (To Kill a Mockingbird, pg. 60).

The third reason Scout should not be punished for crawling under the Radley fence is she honored a friend. Boo had been watching Scout, Jem, and Dill as they played and went on their little escapades (*To Kill a Mockingbird*, pg. 28). He had also been leaving not a few trinkets and toys in the knothole of a neighborhood tree, all gifts for Jem and Scout. Boo left these trinkets until you, Nathan, sealed up the hole, preventing any future gift-giving. A just person would not punish the brave soul who was visiting her friend.

Some say the defense's argument that Scout obeyed Atticus is inadequate because Atticus told her to stay away from the Radleys, not to crawl under their fence. While it is true that Atticus gave her those instructions, they conflicted with his other instruction to stay with Jem. She obeyed the most recent command, after trying to dissuade Jem from going himself. Some say the defense's argument that Jem compelled Scout is inadequate because one is not compelled by name-calling. While it may be true that some people are not compelled by name-calling, Scout knew the name-calling carried with it other, more deleterious consequences. Thus, the prosecution's attack on the defense's case is insufficient.

Scout should not be punished for crawling under the Radley fence because Jem compelled her, she obeyed Atticus, and she honored Boo. Boo is an innocent and good person, who was friendly and kind to Scout. By acquitting Scout, you ensure that Boo will have a friend and even that other neighbors will begin accepting him as part of the community.

Judicial Address Seven: Sample Essay A

Review
Erotema and hypophora

Whether Brutus should be punished for the murder of Julius Caesar

It is true that Brutus appears to be an honorable and wise man, but, hard as it is to accept, he was a cruel assassin. Prior to the Ides of March, Cassius had conspired to kill Caesar, but he needed the help of a highly respected comrade. They knew they needed Brutus, to whom Cassius and a number of co-conspirators subtly presented his plan. Through his efforts, Brutus was persuaded. The following morning, the whole faction went to Pompey's Theater, where the Senate was meeting. There Brutus, Cassius, and the conspirators confronted Caesar, and Brutus had to decide whether to fulfill the plan and execute the ruler of Rome. What do you think he did?

Everyone agrees that Brutus killed Caesar. While some believe Brutus should not be punished for murdering Caesar, others believe he should. Brutus should be punished for three reasons: the evidence of Brutus' own words, the demands of the law, and the absence of a justification.

The first reason Brutus should be punished for murdering Caesar is the evidence of Brutus' own words. After the murder, did Brutus mount the rostrum and proclaim to the Roman people that he and the other conspirators had killed Caesar? Yes, yes he did. He was shameless in his confession, so much so that he brazenly allowed Antony to speak after him, thinking people would overlook his act because of his character. He was wrong. His confession should lead to his punishment.

The second reason Brutus should be punished for murdering Caesar is the demands of the law. He broke the law that underlies every society: You must not murder, and you must especially not murder your rulers. The law of nature prohibits murder, and Roman law going back to the *mos maiorum* had pronounced not the weakest penalties for such an evil deed.

The third reason Brutus should be punished for murdering Caesar is the absence of a justification. Brutus had no excuse for his action, because he did it freely, without accident or compulsion. He had motive: to be remembered as a hero like his ancestor. But he had no justification for his action because there is no higher law to which a murderer can appeal. Ten million tongues could not explain this horrific crime, the worst in all of world history.

Some people say Brutus should not be punished for murdering Caesar because he did keep a higher law: the preservation of the Roman Republic. Brutus' duty to the Republic, however, was as false as his honor. His love of glory led him into folly and his desire for power led to the collapse of the Republic. The idea that the Republic could be preserved by murdering its ruler is not an appeal to a higher law but the vain ravings of an unbalanced man.

Others say Brutus should not be punished for murdering Caesar because the murder prevented greater harms. It is hard to imagine a worse harm than the ensuing civil war, the slaughter of Roman armies, citizens, and even illustrious senators like Cicero, and the end of the Republic for which Brutus claimed he was fighting.

Neither of these arguments–that Brutus kept a higher law or that he prevented greater harms–justify Brutus' actions.

Brutus should be punished for murdering Caesar because of the evidence of Brutus' sword, the demands of the law, and the absence of justification. Cicero would be indignant if the republic were to collapse into civil war should Brutus get away with the assassination.

Judicial Address Seven: Sample Address B

Audience: Nathan Radley

Whether Scout should be punished for trespassing

Boo is an innocent and good person, but this is exactly the reason why Scout should not be punished. That night, Atticus had left Scout in Jem's care. Jem and Dill were busy bragging about their bravery to each other and daring each other to touch the Radley house. When Jem and Dill acted on each other's dares, Scout was dragged along to the Radley house.

Everyone agrees that trespassing is illegal. Some say Scout should be punished for crawling under the Radley fence, and others say she should not. Scout should not be punished for crawling under the Radley fence for three reasons: Jem compelled her, she obeyed Atticus, and she honored a friend.

The first reason Scout should not be punished for crawling under the Radley fence is that Jem compelled her. Wasn't Jem Scout's older brother? Yes. Wasn't Jem supposed to be watching her? Yes. He, however, was busy daring Dill and wanted to go to the Radley house to prove his bravery. Scout tried to talk them out of it, but Jem and Dill simply made fun of her for acting like a girl (*To Kill a Mockingbird*, pg. 60). This helps us to see that Scout went against her will.

The second reason Scout should not be punished for crawling under the Radley fence is Atticus told her to stay with Jem. As above, Scout was obligated to remain with Jem. While it may appear that Scout was disobeying Atticus, who told her to leave the Radleys alone, Scout was actually obeying Atticus, who told her to stay with Jem. Scout had to choose between two conflicting commands. She chose the most recent one and obeyed it. I now realize that she "had no option but to join them" (*To Kill a Mockingbird*, pg. 60).

The third reason Scout should not be punished for crawling under the Radley fence is that she honored a friend. Boo had been watching Scout, Jem, and Dill as they played and went on their little escapades (*To Kill a Mockingbird*, pg. 28). He had also been leaving little trinkets and toys in the knothole of a neighborhood tree, all gifts for Jem and Scout. Boo left these trinkets until you, Nathan, sealed up the hole, preventing any future gift-giving. Would you punish the brave soul for visiting her friend?

Some say the defense's argument that Scout obeyed Atticus is inadequate because Atticus told her to stay away from the Radleys, not to crawl under their fence. While it is true that Atticus gave her those instructions, they conflicted with his other instruction to stay with Jem. She obeyed the most recent command, after trying to dissuade Jem from going himself. Some say the defense's argument that Jem compelled Scout is inadequate because one is not compelled by name-calling. While it may be true that some people are not compelled by name-calling, Scout knew the name-calling carried with it other, more deleterious consequences. Thus, the prosecution's attack on the defense's case is insufficient.

Scout should not be punished for crawling under the Radley fence because Jem compelled her, she obeyed Atticus, and she honored Boo. Boo is an innocent and good person, who was friendly and kind to Scout. By acquitting Scout, you ensure that Boo will have a friend and even that other neighbors may begin accepting him as part of the community.

Glossary

Alliteration: Repeating the same beginning consonants in three or more adjacent words

Amplification: An element that increases the impact of an idea in an essay. It can be used with a sentence, a paragraph, or an element of Arrangement, such as thecConclusion. In LTW I, it was used with the conclusion. In LTW II, it is used with the conclusion and with sentences.

An Sit: A special topic that is used to collect evidence to determine whether an act occurred and whether the defendant committed the act.

Anaphora: A scheme in which the same word or phrase is repeated at the beginning of successive phrases, clauses, or sentences

Antithesis: Two contrasting ideas written in a parallel structure.

Apostrophe: Addressing a personified inanimate object, a deceased person, yourself, or an idea

Argument: One of the three main points in the body or case section of a judicial address

Assonance: A scheme in which one vowel sound is repeated in adjacent or closely connected words

Case: The body of the judicial address, made up of the three arguments. In LTW I, this section was referred to as the proof section.

Circumstance: A common topic that describes the actions and events that occur at the same time as but in different locations from the situation of the issue.

Comparison: A common topic. It asks how two terms are similar and different.

Definition: A common topic. It states the limits within which a word has meaning.

Division: A precise statement of the agreement and disagreement between the writer and an opponent.

Epistrophe: A scheme in which the same word or phrase is repeated at the end of successive phrases, clauses, or sentences

Erotema: A trope that asks a question in order to elicit a specific response. It is designed to subtly influence the response the writer wishes to obtain from his audience. In its simplest form, the answer will be either "yes" or "no."

Exordium: The opening of an essay, speech, or address, placed at the beginning of the introduction. Its purpose is to make the audience receptive to reading or listening

Hyperbole: A trope that makes a point by exaggerating an idea to an impossible or unreal proportion

Hypophora: A trope in which a question is asked and then answered afterwards

Justice: A special topic. It asks if the action of issue was right, fair, or appropriate.

Litotes: Emphasizing a point by negating its opposite

Metaphor: A trope that indirectly (i.e., not using "like" or "as") compares two things that are different in kind but that share a similar trait.

Narratio: Narrative; also called a "statement of facts" or "statement of circumstances." It tells a story, with settings, actors, and actions, to inform the reader of circumstances leading up to and causing the action that is the subject of the thesis.

Parallelism: Sentence structure that lines up parts of speech the same way in a series of words, phrases, or clauses

Personification: A trope in which human characteristics are attributed to an inanimate object

Proof: The body of the essay in LTW I or the particular reasons that make up the body of essay in LTW II. The term is replaced by case in the judicial address when referring to the body and by argument when referring to the individual reasons in the body.

Quale Sit: A special topic. It is used to discover why a defendant committed an act and whether the act is justifiable or excusable.

Quid Sit: A special topic used to discover what happened and whether a law was violated.

Refutation: The response to an opposing argument

Relation: A common topic. It lists events or actions that take place before and after the situation of the issue and determines which are causes and which are effects.

Simile: A trope that explicitly compares two things that are different in kind but that similar in some trait

Synecdoche: A trope in which a physical part of a thing is used to represent, or name, the whole thing.

Testimony: A common topic that asks witnesses what they know about the situation or the event.

Appendix Three: Arrangement Templates

Complete Persuasive Essay

I. **Introduction**
   A. Exordium*
   B. Narratio
      1. Situation*
      2. Actions*
   C. Division
      1. Agreement*
      2. Disagreement
         a. Counter-Thesis*
         b. Thesis*
   D. Distribution
      1. Thesis*
      2. Enumeration*
      3. Exposition
         a. Proof I*
         b. Proof II*
         c. Proof III*

II. **Proof**
   A. Proof I*
      1. Support 1*
      2. Support 2*
      3. Support 3*
   B. Proof II*
      1. Support 1*
      2. Support 2*
      3. Support 3*
   C. Proof III*
      1. Support 1*
      2. Support 2*
      3. Support 3*

III. **Refutation**
   A. Counter-Thesis*
   B. Counter-Proof I*
      1. Summary of support for Counter-Proof I*
      2. Inadequacy of Counter-Proof I*
   C. Counter-Proof II*
      1. Summary of support for Counter-Proof II*
      2. Inadequacy of Counter-Proof II*
   D. Summary of Refutation*

IV. **Conclusion**
   A. Thesis*
   B. Summary of Proof
      1. Proof I*
      2. Proof II*
      3. Proof III*
   C. Amplification
      1. To whom it matters*
      2. Why it matters*

Judicial Addresses One

I. **I. Introduction**
- A. Exordium*
- B. Narratio
    1. Cause 1**
    2. Cause 2**
    3. Cause 3**
    4. Situation**
- C. Division
    1. Agreement*
    2. Disagreement
        a. Counter-Thesis*
        b. Thesis*
- D. Distribution
    1. Thesis*
    2. Enumeration*
    3. Exposition
        a. Proof I*
        b. Proof II*
        c. Proof III*

II. **Proof**
- A. Proof I*
    1. Support 1*
    2. Support 2*
    3. Support 3*
- B. Proof II*
    1. Support 1*
    2. Support 2*
    3. Support 3*
- C. Proof III*
    1. Support 1*
    2. Support 2*
    3. Support 3*

III. **Refutation**
- A. Counter-Thesis*
- B. Counter-Proof I*
    1. Summary of support for Counter-Proof I*
    2. Inadequacy of Counter-Proof I*
- C. Counter-Proof II*
    1. Summary of support for Counter-Proof II*
    2. Inadequacy of Counter-Proof II*
- D. Summary of Refutation*

IV. **Conclusion**
- A. Thesis*
- B. Summary of Proof
    1. Proof I*
    2. Proof II*
    3. Proof III*
- C. Amplification
    1. To whom it matters*
    2. Why it matters*

** In previous outlines, you have left the name of the outline point (i.e., Narratio) or replaced the name (i.e., agreement with information). Those that you replace are identified with a single asterix. When you see the double asterix, you will include both the name and your information in the outline point.

<u>Judicial Address Two</u>

I. **Introduction**
   A. Exordium*
   B. Narratio
      1. Cause 1**
      2. Cause 2**
      3. Cause 3**
      4. Situation**
   C. Division
      1. Agreement*
      2. Disagreement
         a. Counter-Thesis*
         b. Thesis*
   D. Distribution
      1. Thesis*
      2. Enumeration*
      3. Exposition
         a. Argument I*
         b. Argument II*
         c. Argument III*

II. **Case**
   A. Argument I*
      1. Support 1*
      2. Support 2*
      3. Support 3*
   B. Argument II*
      1. Support 1*
      2. Support 2*
      3. Support 3*
   C. Argument III*
      1. Support 1*
      2. Support 2*
      3. Support 3*

III. **Refutation**
   A. Counter-Thesis*
   B. Counter-Argument I*
      1. Summary of support for Counter-Argument I*
      2. Inadequacy of Counter-Argument I*
   C. Counter-Argument II*
      1. Summary of support for Counter-Argument II*
      2. Inadequacy of Counter-Argument II*
   D. Summary of Refutation*

IV. **Conclusion**
   A. Thesis*
   B. Summary of Case
      1. Argument I*
      2. Argument II*
      3. Argument III*
   C. Amplification
      1. To whom it matters*
      2. Why it matters*

Judicial Addresses Three through Seven

I. **Introduction**
   A. Kind of Exordium*
   B. Narratio
      1. Cause 1**
      2. Cause 2**
      3. Cause 3**
      4. Situation**
   C. Division
      1. Agreement*
      2. Disagreement
         a. Counter-Thesis*
         b. Thesis*
   D. Distribution
      1. Thesis*
      2. Enumeration*
      3. Exposition
         a. Argument I*
         b. Argument II*
         c. Argument III*

II. **Case**
   A. Argument I*
      1. Support 1*
      2. Support 2*
      3. Support 3*
      4. Kind of Terminating Sentence*
   B. Argument II*
      1. Support 1*
      2. Support 2*
      3. Support 3*
      4. Kind of Terminating Sentence*
   C. Argument III*
      1. Support 1*
      2. Support 2*
      3. Support 3*
      4. Kind of Terminating Sentence*

III. **Refutation**
   A. Counter-Thesis*
   B. Counter-Argument I*
      1. Summary of support for Counter-Argument I*
      2. Inadequacy of Counter-Argument I*
   C. Counter-Argument II*
      1. Summary of support for Counter-Argument II*
      2. Inadequacy of Counter-Argument II*
   D. Summary of Refutation*

IV. **Conclusion**
   A. Thesis*
   B. Summary of Case
      1. Argument I*
      2. Argument II*
      3. Argument III*
   C. Amplification
      1. What does the judge care about?*
      2. How will it be affected?*